FLOURISHING CLASSROOMS

FLOURISHING CLASSROOMS

A Deep Dive into Proactive Wellness for Grades 7–12

Jeff Catania

ROWMAN & LITTLEFIELD
Lanham • Boulder • New York • London

Published by Rowman & Littlefield
An imprint of The Rowman & Littlefield Publishing Group, Inc.
4501 Forbes Boulevard, Suite 200, Lanham, Maryland 20706
www.rowman.com

86-90 Paul Street, London EC2A 4NE, United Kingdom

Copyright © 2023 by Jeff Catania

All rights reserved. No part of this book may be reproduced in any form or by any electronic or mechanical means, including information storage and retrieval systems, without written permission from the publisher, except by a reviewer who may quote passages in a review.

British Library Cataloguing in Publication Information Available

Library of Congress Cataloging-in-Publication Data

Names: Catania, Jeff, 1967– author.
Title: Flourishing classrooms : a deep dive into proactive wellness for grades 7-12 / Jeff Catania.
Description: Lanham : Rowman & Littlefield, [2023] | Includes index. | Summary: "A robust and powerful set of wellness activities (47) for grade 7–12 classrooms of all subjects, organized across ten evidence-based domains of well-being, rooted in positive psychology"— Provided by publisher.
Identifiers: LCCN 2022057504 (print) | LCCN 2022057505 (ebook) | ISBN 9781475867459 (cloth) | ISBN 9781475867466 (paperback) | ISBN 9781475867473 (epub)
Subjects: LCSH: Classroom environment—Psychological aspects. | Well-being—Social aspects. | Middle school students—Mental health. | High school students—Mental health. | Middle school students—Social conditions. | High school students—Social conditions. | Educational psychology.
Classification: LCC LB3013 .C38 2023 (print) | LCC LB3013 (ebook) | DDC 371.102/4—dc23/eng/20221229
LC record available at https://lccn.loc.gov/2022057504
LC ebook record available at https://lccn.loc.gov/2022057505

For Evan, Owen, and Barb—the three stars of my game.

CONTENTS

Preface		ix
Acknowledgments		xv
1	Well-Being Goes to School	1
2	Safety	33
3	Social Well-Being	55
4	Eudaimonia	85
5	Resilience	111
6	Cognitive Well-Being	143
7	Emotional Well-Being	175
8	Environmental Well-Being	203
9	Physical Well-Being	213
10	Spiritual Well-Being	235
11	All is Well	253

Appendix A: Achievements Unlocked   259

Appendix B: Activity Keywords   261

Appendix C: Wellness Is in the Cards   263

Notes   273

Index   293

About the Author   305

PREFACE

Living the Questions of Well-Being

"Have patience with everything unresolved in your heart and love the questions themselves, like locked rooms or books written in a foreign language. Do not seek the answers, which could not be given to you now, because you would not be able to live them. And the point is, to live everything. Live the questions now. Then perhaps someday you will gradually, without even noticing it, live your way into the answers."[1]

—Rainer Maria Rilke

In the midst of a challenging career in education and busy family life, a devastating setback had brought me to a lifetime low. The anguish and shame led me to attend a support group, where I remember sitting down at my first meeting, stomach churning. I barely heard the others speaking as my turn to share approached. When I did talk, the words came with sobs and tears. I eventually trailed to a stop and noticed for the first time a bright-eyed woman sitting quietly next to me. With an unmistakably caring tone, she spoke a question in the silence that marked my watershed between a lifetime low and a life of flourishing:

"*So what makes you well?*"

This question ultimately changed my life. Yet when I first heard it that day, my mind couldn't have been any emptier. I felt what my students must have experienced when I stumped them with a physics problem. I had a clear understanding of all the sad and painful aspects of my life situation. I also excelled at pleasing others. But I had no idea what could make me truly well. For all my privilege and years in school, I hadn't the foggiest clue about what was personally positive, meaningful, or joy-inducing.

After a few moments of stunned silence, I had a magical teaching/learning moment (MTLM)—and my wellness journey began—with a single word bubbling up: *"hiking."*

I did go hiking, which involved more crying, except with trees. But in those woods I also had moments of actual happiness, partly from the exercise, but also from being in beautiful nature. Yoga classes followed, and my first hot class felt better than ten years of martial arts had ever felt. Doing what felt good for me was a balm for my body and soul after years of enduring and striving to please others. My empty wellness basket now contained a single egg of pleasure or *hedonia*, but it sure tasted sweet.

Hiking and yoga connected me with wellness-oriented people, which led me to join a meditation community, take a group course, start therapy, and generally open up. For years I had been socially disconnected, and in that time of need I rapidly cultivated friendships. At the age of forty-five, I rediscovered the richness of having a best friend, and the deliciousness of sharing deeply.

My solo well-being journey became collaborative, with support from people who freely shared their love and experience. I could now include *social well-being* in my repertoire.

As my analytical ways awkwardly shifted over on the bench to make space for a social-emotional teammate, my career also shifted. At the time I had moved from the classroom to lead district programs in math, e-learning, and technology. I was proud of this work but also attached to it. When the superintendent told me in my year of devastation I would be switching roles, I resisted. My self-worth was tied to contributing and engaging analytically, and now I would have to look for new sources of *cognitive well-being*.

It turned out in the end, for with devastation comes at least one gift: the opportunity to rebuild anew. The next years became the most rewarding of my career as I supported applied programs, launched a staff and student mindfulness initiative, led the district Restorative Practices team, and became an unofficial well-being champion. When the support group facilitator stepped down and asked me to take over, I did. Technology had been a comfort zone, and these head-to-heart flip-flops generated growth and meaning like never before. My wellness capacities swelled with a newfound sense of growth and purpose: the domain of *eudaimonia*.

What surprised me most was discovering how the adversity I was facing, combined with the opportunities and privileges I had, actually *contributed* to well-being. I had taken two sick days off in the first twenty years of my career but took twenty off in the next two. While commuting one day during those two years, waiting behind a line of cars, some awful and familiar triggers began to loop inside me. As I grimly debated whether to head home, or continue to work and repress, I had another MTLM.

A course I was taking at the time had suggested focusing on the physical experience of being triggered and not the thoughts. I took a breath and tried this. For a whole minute, I just tried to feel my body, which was so new for me that my brain paused in confusion. The mental stress vanished, and I stayed with a roiling feeling in my chest. It was only mildly uncomfortable, and far better than the torturous thoughts. I had realized a brand-new form of wellness: the presence and poignancy of staying with difficulty rather than avoiding it. As the experience faded, the traffic magically dissolved, and I turned into work, beaming at the discovery of this newfound superpower and wellness domain: *resilience* in the face of adversity.

Discovering wellness felt like a miracle, and I kept asking myself why I hadn't learned any of these lessons in school. Education prepared me for life but not for living it well. Schools had changed little since I was a student, continuing their focus on academic knowledge and skills. I realized the vast institution of education was missing a golden opportunity: to explicitly teach students the full spectrum of well-being domains.

My self-taught well-being journey then took a deeper turn. I joined an open-hearted spiritual group and intensified my other well-being practices like mindfulness. Previously fleeting states of relaxation and acceptance became more continual. Healthy actions that had formerly punctuated a life of misery began to string together into an ongoing thriving.

None of it resembled any class in school I had ever taken, yet I was learning and growing like never before. I saw how I wasn't alone in suffering or healing: that everyone had *something*. I saw how unhealed emotional wounds could hamper people for years. I also saw how flourishing was neither mysterious nor unattainable. Ultimately, in the ups and downs and ups again, a peak came into view. I had a monumental experience of well-being that changed me forever.

Five seasons after that support group meeting, lying prone at the end of an otherwise typical yoga class, an unusually deep and vast relief swept through me. Gratitude was there, but also love and compassion. I had been feeling horrible for most of the past year, so this ought to have felt surprising, but the feeling was absolutely natural and easy—a pure and endless love that seemingly emanated from everywhere.

As the blissful love expanded, I walked out of the studio not in a trance but with an utter clarity that *love is all there is.* For two weeks I lived in a state of profound grace and compassion. Life flowed effortlessly as my self-referential thoughts, background anxiety, and all forms of stress had vanished. The only constant was a seemingly eternal ocean of peaceful love and a feeling of being in seamless harmony with all life and the planet.

In this state, relationships blossomed—including with strangers—as I could sense people's emotional states and form instant connections. The "problems" of my life no longer felt problematic but with clear and harmonious paths forward issuing from a deep well of love. This elevated state eventually faded, but my life was transformed forever. The experience of absolute peace, joy, and love left no doubt that this was my truest nature—a pure expression of well-being.

By this time I certainly hadn't found all the answers, but I was at least asking some different questions, starting with the one asked of me: *what makes you well?* And as I lived these questions—gradually, without even noticing it—I began to live my way into some answers.

- If success is chasing happiness, wealth, and status, then why does that feel so unwell?

- Is well-being simply the absence of illness, is it mental health, or something else entirely?
- Is baseline wellness fixed for life, or are there ways to change it?
- How can well-being be integrated with learning in classrooms and schools?
- How can wellness be social: developed collaboratively and shared for the greater good?
- Can the school community and world beyond benefit from classroom well-being?
- Could the ultimate aim of public education shift to a union of learning and well-being?

This book offers responses to these questions, and an invitation to live the questions in your own classrooms, schools, and lives. Living the questions of well-being benefits students, teachers, and everyone. We don't thrive and flourish alone, but always and together as one.

ACKNOWLEDGMENTS*

"A teacher affects eternity."[1]

—Henry Brooks Adams

Bless you Cate Roberts, for turning in your auditorium seat to my fifteen-year-old self, moments after a poet had stunned every English class in the school to silence with a verse, and whispering so I alone could hear, *"you* could write like *that."*

My deepest gratitude, and great admiration, goes to beloved colleagues, experts, family, friends, leaders, teachers, and wellness champions (choose three or more each of you) who loved this book—and me personally—to wholeness. You are in these words and in my heart: Wendy Redfearn, Sheri Hill, Rebecca Reble, Melissa De Benedetti, Meg Merwart, Meg Carey, Laura Smallbone, Kelly Hoey, Karen Schindler, Karamjit Sangha-Bosland, Jennie Akse-Kelly, Ginny Catania, Damian Cooper, Barb Noack, Ashtyn Ford, and Ardith Dean.

I am indebted, and give huge props, to Liza Crawford, Lisa Mackenzie, Kelly Judge, and Holly Moniz: teachers who pioneered classroom well-being long before it was a thing, and gave freely of their prep time to review a chapter—or three.

In defiance of class lists everywhere, given in reverse alphabetical order by first name.

A district-level thank you to Tali Aikenhead, Michelle McCann, and Nicole Hagley, who contributed chapter guidance in their particular areas of expertise and do the same every day for teachers in the many schools they support.

A two-minute hug to Anne Louise Carney, for asking the question that started it all.

To every "teacher" who shaped me, whether schoolteachers or not, you all affected eternity, and you all have my sincere appreciation and love.

1

WELL-BEING GOES TO SCHOOL

"If we are to reach real peace in the world, we shall have to begin with the children."

—Mahatma Gandhi

Questions of well-being aren't just personal. They lie at the core of a flurry of worldwide innovations in human thriving in governments and non-governmental organizations:

- Many countries (including Bolivia, Ecuador, Namibia, New Zealand, the United Kingdom, and the United Arab Emirates) are using well-being indicators to set policy, make budgets, and measure domestic progress.
- The Social Progress Index[1] and World Happiness Report[2] are redefining success, balancing economic factors with health, freedom, equity, and other wellness factors.
- The United Nations prioritizes wellness in their suite of Sustainable Development Goals.[3] But what about education? While wellness is eclipsing economic gain as a primary driver worldwide, it has largely been marked absent from class in schools.

The Programme for International Student Assessment (PISA) reflects this broader neglect, though with pockets of promise. Every three years, fifteen-years-olds around the world take tests set by PISA. Much attention is paid to the rankings of nearly one hundred countries who have participated since 2000. The media sorts scores in reading, math, and science, so tiny gains can be proclaimed or losses lamented. Yet such comparisons have little meaning, and calls to raise the bar have contributed to a harmful proliferation of over-amped curricula and high-stakes testing. Most deeply, they expose an inherent bias for academic performance and its contribution to economic development, over well-being.

The headlines rarely tell the story of the well-being data which PISA has collected since 2015 around belonging, life satisfaction and meaning.[4] In 2018, only 67 percent of students around the world reported being satisfied with their lives—a (big) drop of 5 percent from 2015. To put this in perspective, the mean performance in reading, math, and science has not changed appreciably in two decades. More revealing, the three greatest declines in satisfaction were not in poorer countries but in the United Kingdom, Japan, and the United States. Only one country in the entire world, South Korea, has had any significant increase in life satisfaction since 2015.

Some countries won't have access to PISA well-being data for their students since the wellness questionnaire is optional, unlike academics. But the data collected illuminates a range of student well-being needs worldwide, spanning many domains of well-being:

- Almost a quarter of students reported being bullied at least a few times a month.
- Girls have a greater fear of failure than boys, even when outperforming them significantly, and they are more likely than boys to feel sad in every country in the world.
- More than half of students feel very anxious, even when well-prepared for a test.
- One in three students feel their lives lack meaning or purpose.

These are disturbing findings, and a clarion call for schools to focus on well-being.

The good news is that well-being *is* making its way to school in places, showing up on everything from classroom lesson plans to district long-range plans to curriculum documents. Some early years teachers are inserting wellness into their routines with strategies like "Wellness Wednesdays" or break bins. While these timeouts from the curriculum look more like a break from learning rather than a way of learning, they are vital. Dedicated time for wellness not only benefits students but validates practices of well-being across the entire school community.

In school districts and at the district and governmental levels, formal programs for mindfulness, social-emotional learning, and resilience are proliferating.[5] The curriculum itself is also evolving, with well-being written into formal standards and expectations. Subjects like the arts, career studies, equity studies, and physical and health education already include numerous wellness outcomes, but other subjects are joining in. In Ontario, Canada, even Grade 9 mathematics has social-emotional learning as its very first strand, *to be included in classroom instruction.*[6]

Whether mandatory or not, teachers need well-being activities suitable for any subject area. They also need ways to *integrate* well-being into the fabric of everyday teaching and learning, making it seamless with instruction and assessment. When well-being permeates learning, rather than interrupting it, the two become synergistic and sustainable, not a tradeoff.

Leona, a second-year teacher, felt like all she ever did was mark. When she gave back tests and assignments, her students would ignore her written feedback and skip to the score at the top. Staring at a stack of unmarked quizzes one day, she decided to get students involved in self-assessment. As she coached them in understanding success criteria, and self-assessing as they learned, they eventually began co-creating criteria, and rubrics as well. Leona had intended to boost engagement, but achievement and well-being also climbed as students learned to recognize their own success and feel more like active agents in it.

While grade 1–6 teachers have been early adopters of well-being practices, down the hall and across the street in grades 7 and up, well-being is largely new territory.[7] Cohorts of tweens and teens, who have pressing well-being needs, are lucky if they have a wellness pioneer as a teacher. These students are at a ripe age to explore mature aspects of well-being, yet most of them will have to find wellness elsewhere: at home or in extracurriculars.

Grade 7–12 classrooms also need wellness love, along with ways to share that well-being across their schools, with their families, and in the broader school community. Teachers are also members of those classrooms, and so their personal wellness is vital in itself, and to support wellness in others. Teacher training programs are only beginning to understand this need. The resulting picture is one of an entire educational community looking to come home to wellness.

"A child belongs not to one parent or home" is a proverb in Kihaya (a Tanzanian language) acknowledging that it takes a village to raise a child. Making well-being communal rather than personal shares the load and helps everyone thrive. Teachers who focus on student needs (sometimes at their own expense) can now discover how their own well-being is correlated to student wellness, and vice versa. School districts choosing between student or employee wellness can now take a holistic approach.

If wellness efforts prioritize one group over another, they are ultimately constrained. Classrooms benefit most when students and staff thrive together, meaning teachers need to benefit from well-being activity. Educators accustomed to watching and supporting students in learning need to evolve their role to become active participants with young people in well-being.

This whole-village approach widens impact, provides crucial adult modeling, and reflects the symbiosis between personal, community, and global well-being.[8] This social dynamic in well-being is all-powerful, for as one part of a social network thrives, that wellness inevitably spreads. When well-being is a collective endeavor, self-care/love becomes all-care/love. This book supports a whole-village approach: providing grade 7–12 wellness activities for students and teachers (both add-on and integrated), plus ways to share wellness beyond the classroom.

So while the world, and the world of education, learns to embrace well-being, consider yourself fortunate if your teacher taught wellness in some way. And if, as a teacher, you now take this opportunity to offer well-being to your own students, consider yourself even more fortunate. For nothing is lost in the giving of wellness, as it enriches young lives, our own lives, and the lives of everyone we touch.

HEADING UPSTREAM: FROM NEGATIVITY BIAS TO POSITIVE PSYCHOLOGY

> "There are a thousand hacking at the branches of evil to one who is striking at the root."
>
> —Henry David Thoreau

As well-being is being promoted for its own sake, the term *mental health* (degree of cognitive, emotional, or psychological well-being) is used widely. With one in six youth living with a mental illness (disturbances in thoughts, feelings, or perceptions severe enough to affect day-to-day functioning), it's understandable that this term is prominent:

- Almost half of U.S. children have experienced at least one adverse childhood experience (trauma such as abuse or growing up with a caregiver struggling with addiction), and one in ten children have experienced three or more, putting them at high risk.[9]
- Rates of depression, anxiety, and stress in youth are at alarmingly high levels and correlated with behavior problems in school.[10]
- A worldwide pandemic has had major physical, economic, and psychosocial impacts[11] (including a more isolated and sedentary lifestyle) for students and their families.[12]

These are pressing challenges, and most educators would naturally prioritize them. However, focusing on disorder alone becomes less about wellness and more about recovering from unwellness. At an extreme, hacking at the branches will never get to the root of the issue.

It's tempting to focus on problems. Most people give more mental significance to negative events.[13] Even the researchers themselves who first classified well-being domains, started with depression and anxiety rather than a direct sense of wellness itself.[14] So it's understandable that many school districts focus on reacting to problems, rather than developing wellness proactively. But the result means less progress in positive domains of proactive well-being that could prevent many of these issues in the first place.

Even where a proactive well-being initiative exists, it is often outnumbered by programs and protocols rooted in problems. Anti-bullying, violent threat response, harassment policies, suicide intervention, mental health first aid, and ongoing discipline and suspensions can be lifesavers, but why do so many students need saving? Even more proactive programs (such as Restorative Practices or Collaborative Problem Solving) are still rooted in a reaction to incidents or challenging behaviors, rather than proactive well-being that gets at the heart of the matter.

In 1972, Irving Zola described a health care parable that exemplifies this dilemma.[15] You are standing on the shore of a swiftly flowing river with a friend and notice a child drowning in the water. You jump in and pull them ashore, only to hear the cry of another child floating by.

Your friend jumps in to rescue the second child, but then there is another child, and another, all flailing in the river. As you both rush to save drowning kids, your friend suddenly quits, climbs up the bank, and runs away. "What are you doing?" you yell. Your friend shouts back, "I'm going upstream, to find out who the heck is throwing these kids in the water!"

What lies upstream is a golden opportunity to thrive positively in every domain of well-being, widening out from a focus on disorder and mental health alone. What lies upstream is a proactive, multidimensional well-being that benefits everyone: not just students, not just staff, and not just those in crisis. To move upstream is to recognize the centrality of well-being in human thriving and flourishing, regardless of whether a preexisting problem or trauma exists. Well-being no longer needs to be justified by its opposite.

Policy makers, researchers, and educators alike are now exploring this positive frame in addition to tackling disorder.[16] The approaches in this book are based in positive psychology to cultivate positive human traits of thriving, not just deal with what's gone wrong.[17] Being on the plus side offers benefits for every domain of well-being in a foundational way. A 2016 report on positive psychology "calls for as much focus on strength as on weakness, as much interest in building the best things in life as in repairing the worst, and as much attention to fulfilling the lives of healthy people as to healing the wounds of the distressed."[18]

There is still a need for mental health initiatives, clinicians, and trauma-informed classrooms to help students at risk. In addition, historic and ongoing systems of oppression must be dismantled to have any foundation for well-being. Chapter 2, "Safety—Essential Needs and

Freedoms," explores these areas. But wellness efforts must balance the addressing of challenges with the development of positive thriving for its own sake. Martin Seligman, a founder of positive psychology, recognized this: "Curing the negatives does not produce the positives."[19] Indeed, those positives can avoid many of those challenges in the first place.

A move upstream toward proactive well-being can also shift the negativity bias of an entire student generation. This doesn't mean ignoring what's wrong but placing a primary focus on the positive domains of well-being. These include the domains associated with mental health and resilience, but also every other domain. The domain of resilience (p. 111) reflects the emergence of well-being in education: rooted in challenge but turning upstream toward thriving.

The Domains of Well-Being

So if mental health is one aspect of well-being, what are the other domains? The research community has identified a rainbow of well-being domains with strikingly similar findings:

- A large-scale study identified social connectedness as the number one domain, followed by physical well-being, resilience, emotional/mental health, meaning, and more.[20]
- A large-scale study of flourishing found well-being to be multidimensional, including engagement, emotional stability, meaning, positive relationships, and resilience.[21]
- Taxonomies identified by Seligman and Mihaly Csikszentmihalyi (the psychologist who originally studied flow) reaffirm a spectrum of domains including engagement, flow, meaning, positive emotional experiences, and relationships.[22]
- Wellness and flourishing researchers Ryff[23] and Keyes[24] came up with similar terms: emotional well-being (hedonia), positive relations, psychological/social well-being (eudaimonia), and purpose.

The implication of all this for schools is to take a much broader—and *deeper*—view of wellness than mental health alone. Only a comprehensive approach to well-being can produce correspondingly wholehearted, whole-bodied, whole-minded, and whole-spirited graduates.

Comprehensive well-being requires classroom activities and school-wide extensions that span a complete spectrum of domains, all of which are presented as chapters in this book:

- *Safety: Essential Needs and Freedoms* highlights basic needs, freedom from harm, and plain old freedom as a foundation on which to build other domains.
- *Social Well-Being: Relationships, Community, and Belonging* explores the cardinal domain of human connection for wellness individually and in groups.
- *Eudaimonia: Meaning, Excellence, Growth, and Authenticity* combines our sense of self, purpose, growth, and achievement as related routes to self-actualized well-being.
- *Resilience: Transforming Challenge into Thriving* explores this surprisingly vital capacity to find wellness, growth, and even flow, in adversity.
- *Cognitive Well-Being: Mental and Intellectual Health* addresses the familiar area of mental health but also optimal experience and mindful engagement with life.
- *Emotional Well-Being: Hedonia and Beyond* starts with feeling good and adds on ways to expand and enrich our emotional world, rewiring the heart for optimal well-being.
- *Environmental Well-Being: Wellness with the Natural World* cultivates well-being within the vital connection to nature, in the context of the current environmental crisis.
- *Physical Well-Being: Healthy Bodies, Balanced Lifestyles* bolsters the familiar areas of diet, sleep, exercise, and healthy behaviors in the backdrop of a youth health epidemic.
- *Spiritual Well-Being: Transcendence, Union, and Peace* intersects with every other domain, inviting a merging of the universal with our embodied, everyday life.

In this chapter sequence, safety is presented first, with social well-being next as a primary domain of well-being. Eudaimonia and resilience follow as potent and enduring (if less familiar) sources of wellness. The next five chapters present classic domains of human thriving, though less emphasis is placed on physical health since it is addressed well in many schools. Other vital domains of sexual, financial, or vocational well-being also find support in health classes, financial literacy, and cooperative education, careers, or experiential learning programs.

While a holistic approach is most likely to boost overall wellness, teachers and students may spend more time in some domains over others. Comfort may guide this, but a willingness to stretch and grow comfort zones is key to well-being. Fortunately, the domains are strongly interconnected, so developing any one grows them all. Working in every domain is powerfully, mutually, reinforcing for the well-being of every stakeholder, indeed for all life and the planet.

Using This Book

> "Begin doing what you want to do now. We are not living in eternity. We have only this moment, shining like a star in our hand and melting like a snowflake."
>
> —Francis Bacon

Flourishing Classrooms supports grade 7–12 educators in the development and sharing of well-being by employing several key features. These components provide a toolkit for educators to cultivate well-being across the school community in a synergistic way.

1. *Full spectrum of positive, proactive well-being domains* by chapter, providing a balanced, holistic approach to well-being. Foundational activities are shown as "Main Moves."
2. *Well-being activities* suited for grade 7–12 classrooms that benefit students, teachers, and the school community. Each activity begins with a preamble, one-line summary, and required time and trust level (see p. 37). Detailed step-by-step instructions follow, including teacher prompts, safety considerations, and the features outlined below:
   a. *Integration strategies* infuse daily classroom routines of teaching, learning, assessment, and homework with well-being.
   b. *Schoolwide extensions* offer options to share and scale wellness schoolwide.

c. *Lifeplay* (a twist on homework) invites students and staff to playfully explore well-being throughout their lives beyond school.
   d. *Keywords* tag every activity with their related domains(s) and other characteristics such as "mindfulness," "prep-free," or "lifeplay." An index (p. 293) references every activity and supplementary resource by keyword.
3. *Supplementaries* offer additional wellness ideas that are shorter, simpler, safer, and/or easily searchable online, to complement more detailed chapter activities. While presented in brief, many of these strategies can be explored to great depth. The search terms provided point to starting points to find out more.
4. *Shareable cards* (see p. 263) are a subset of activities suitable for sharing in the broader school community, presented in a shareable card size for photo sharing or copying.

With so many domains, activities, and more in a potentially all-new area, it's natural for educators to feel over their heads. But with well-being, less can be more. Relax, and start easy. Rather than jamming more into plans, discern what can be replaced, removed, or transformed.

Kelly Judge is a high school drama teacher and department head who for decades has led workshops for new and preservice teachers. Teachers love her creative wellness activities, but they wonder how they can fit them into packed courses. Kelly shares, "My greatest joy is showing them how they can actually do both at the same time—by integrating well-being into their curriculum—and watching their faces light up."

Even experienced teachers may feel stretched to explore well-being deeply with certain classes. Kindness and patience will allow students and teachers to grow into the qualities and practices that can spark a synergistic blaze of flourishing. To support a broad spectrum of teachers and students, a variety of approaches to the book are possible:

- *Those who struggle with well-being* may read the introduction in full, try some simpler supplements, then venture into activities and domains as comfort and capacity builds.
- *Those newer to well-being* may read through the introduction, then the chapters, but not necessarily all chapter activities. In class, use activities with the keyword "short-'n'-safe" (see p. 262) or supple-

ments. The domains are ordered such that anyone who follows them can develop a safe and powerful classroom wellness practice.
- *Those with some previous well-being experience* could start with the introduction, safety, and social well-being domains, and explore others according to classroom needs or personal interests. All activities provide a requisite level of trust, so preexisting classroom capacity can be taken into account. In any case, exploring any one domain will naturally lead to the others due to their strong interconnection.
- *Well-being innovators or wellness early adopters with deeper experience* could check over safety, then focus on domains that feel most intriguing. They may then jump into activities and supplements by keyword (see indexes p. 293) according to specific needs.

All readers are encouraged to explore the shareable cards (see p. 263), since community well-being is a key factor in personal well-being, and vice versa.

However prepared a teacher may feel to explore wellness with students, the nature of wellness work leads to some final implications for all grade 7–12 educators:

- *Well-being is rooted in safety* so begin with this all-important domain to ensure future wellness efforts (which will ideally span multiple domains) can take hold and grow.
- *Well-being is experiential* so try some activities before sharing them to build clarity and authenticity. Also present some activities fresh (and let students know) to model courage and a growth mindset. Most of all, *participate* in wellness activities with the class.
- *Well-being is collective* so look for schoolwide extensions, lifeplay, and shareable cards to spread wellness throughout social networks in and out of school. As wellness is developed in students and teachers, it will naturally spread to families, colleagues, and beyond, creating a supportive network of well-being that benefits everyone.
- *Well-being is integrated* so use some of the integration strategies to infuse everyday classroom life with wellness, in addition to add-on

strategies. Most activities can be split up over multiple days to flexibly use smaller chunks of classroom time.
- *Well-being is personal* so just *be you* in practicing and sharing wellness. Let your unique energy, intuition, and creativity guide and shape the sharing. Consider your own wellness needs along with those of students, as the activities benefit adults and youth alike.

Above all, relax and enjoy the well-being voyage. The chapter domains of this book are validated by research, interdependent, rooted in positive, proactive wellness, and universal in their benefit to individuals and groups. Most compellingly, they also correlate to learning itself, allowing educators to put well-being in its rightful place at the very heart of human development—the core mission of schools.[25]

Well Wishes: Questions of Living

"Everything is moving toward its place of wholeness. Befriending life requires that we listen for that potential which is trying to actualize itself over time. It will be there whether we are listening to a tree, a person, an organization, or a society. Everything has a deep dream of itself and its fulfillment."[26]

—Rachel Naomi Remen

Who are you?
What is your deepest dream?
Is it for fulfillment in a life of well-being?
Does it include your own world, and ours together?
Do you see the children, school, and trees in the yard as one?
Can we dream together of teaching students all the facets of well-being?
What if learning and well-being was a union, with neither supplanting the other?
Could this union become the ultimate dream of all teachers, of all schools?
What if this dream led all life to an ocean of well-being together?
If we dive in together, can we transcend separateness?
Can it all be a single deep dream of union?
What is your deepest dream?
Who are you?

Key Messages

- Well-being is an emerging priority all over the world, including in education.
- Wellness in the classroom can be a break from learning and also integrated with learning.
- Members of communities thrive together, as wellness is shared in social networks.
- A proactive, positive approach to well-being balances the tendency to focus on problems.
- Exploring multiple domains supports a comprehensive, holistic approach to well-being.
- Use chapter activities, supplementaries, and shareable cards, along with the options for integration, lifeplay, and schoolwide sharing, to best foster communal well-being.
- Multiple pathways through the book are available based on teacher readiness.
- Start with safety, participate as a teacher, and make wellness your own.

INTRODUCTORY ACTIVITIES

Debriefing Anything: Mining for Meaning (Main Move)

"Life can only be understood backwards; but it must be lived forwards."

—Søren Kierkegaard

A life of well-being is a life well lived: its flavor tasted vividly and deeply in a wide-open heart. As experiences warm and soften us, they also seep into our cracks, letting in some light. On those rare and beautiful peak experiences when we fully open, there can be a tipping into absolute peace, heart-splitting grief, or pure love. We are then transformed, carrying a new whole-heartedness or aliveness into the rest of our lives.

For many people however, this is not the norm. Social or familial conditioning typically leans toward being more closed rather than open. Eventually, the accumulation of armor, walls, masks, and numbing can block out life and make change difficult. With these blockages, life's experiences don't touch us to the core—or don't touch us at all.

Debriefing experiences in a trusted group can help dissolve these barriers and let well-being permeate deeply. After an experience prepares our ground, the debrief helps it work its way inward where buried healing, joy, or insight can be found. Learning when to open up, and with whom, is a vital wellness skill that will also help students in life beyond school.

While the word debrief implies a post-experience questioning, it is also important to *pre*-brief, activating prior well-being knowledge and capacities. What is most beneficial is to watch for magical teaching/learning moments (MTLMs) *during* an activity in order to pause and debrief on the fly.

In a senior class activity, Mx. Pereira secretly gave students different animal cards and asked them to form groups without using words (see p. 106). As the teens clued in that they could make sounds and gestures, they began to form into like-species groups. Emily, a horse, was searching in vain for other horses, but she didn't realize her card had no match. Her friend Makayla had already joined the squirrel group but noticed Emily's distress. Makayla stepped out in the bustle of students, took Emily by the arm, and brought a horse into the squirrel nest. This went unnoticed by the class, and so Mx. Pereira paused the activity to unpack the motivation, beauty, and subtle social dynamics behind Makayla's gesture of inclusion.

Let the duration of the debrief be flexible, in proportion to the significance of the experience and richness of the discussion. A short but powerful experience may require more debriefing, to find interesting forks in the dialogue. The "questions to debrief anything" (table 1.1) are open-ended to support this widening of perspectives, impact, and meaning.

Whatever the timing or subject of a debrief, taking time to reflect has many benefits:

- Giving thoughts and feelings additional time and space to surface.
- Sharing personal wellness insights that may germinate in others.
- Confirming we are not alone while celebrating uniqueness.

- Exploring questions and challenges with the group's support and collective wisdom.
- Talking about any discomfort that may have surfaced during an experience.
- Feeling elevation from the witnessing of moral beauty in group interaction.
- Finding connections together that make meaning of life's experiences.

Keep in mind these are *potential* benefits: not all debriefs will be meaningful or magical. Some may be comical or feel downright flat. That's okay. It just means that nothing came up, students are still processing, or perhaps don't wish to share. All these scenarios are perfectly fine.

Sometimes debriefs are not necessary or beneficial. Some experiences may not feel significant enough to be discussed, while others may be so significant that a debrief could only lessen them.

This activity gives teachers a set of universal debrief questions (loosely based on Restorative Practices questions) and a framework to debrief any experience.[27] Use these questions and the process below to explore the power and potential of debriefs and see what meaning can be unearthed in the classroom.

> **Summary**: Debrief any classroom experience by sharing thoughts, feelings, and more.
> **Time**: 1–15 minutes
> **Trust Required**: Varies
>
> 1. *Prep* (optional): Most debriefs are best held as freeform discussions, without preplanning what questions will be asked, although it may be important to scaffold for English language learners by giving prompts ahead of time or have table 1.1 printed and handy.
> 2. *Debrief Stages*: Consider using a series of debrief options such as *personal reflection (think), partner talk (pair), groups of 4 (square), whole group (share),* and *personal writing (journal).* A staged debrief slows the reflection process, giving

each participant time to find connections and meaning for themselves and with others.
3. *Notice Moments*: During any classroom experience, watch for magical teaching/learning moments (MTLMs) and pause to debrief, whether during or after the activity.
4. *Debrief*: Invite students to share using the questions below. Sharing may be sequential (see p. 61) but more often evolves organically. These questions are broad enough to use with any activity or domain of wellness. Use some, all, or none of them according to your intuition and discretion. Also discern when a totally different question (usually in a MTLM) could take a group deeply into the heart of *their* experience of *the* experience.

Table 1.1. Questions to Debrief Anything

During Experience	After Experience	Intended Responses
What is happening?	What happened?	Sensory impressions of the experience: what was seen or heard without other commentary.
What are you thinking?	What were you thinking?	Thoughts about the experience: delving into the cognitive domain.
What are you feeling?	What were you feeling?	Feelings about the experience: delving into the emotional domain.
What is the impact?	What was the impact?	Impacts of the experience on self, perceived impacts on others, groups, situations, property, the environment, etc.
Is there any meaning, growth, or connection to find in this?		Mining the experience for eudaimonic aspects of meaning and growth, as well as connections to school or life.
What *could* change, in a good way?		Ideas for positive changes that could bring deeper wellness to the activity, a situation, one's personal self, or others.

5. *Safety*: The trust level required for a debrief is proportional to the challenge and sensitivity of activity. More potent experiences can penetrate more deeply, but require a correspond-

ing depth of group trust, relationships, and grace. Classroom agreements and other safety strategies in the next chapter will help build community for deeper debriefs. Depth of student sharing will grow in proportion to classroom trust, so give students the right to participate or pass during a debrief, and sense when to offer a private or anonymous debrief option. Also keep in mind some may want to debrief with a specific friend, trusted adult, or other resource. Encourage and allow what works for students.

6. *Integration Strategy*: Teachers debrief learning experiences constantly, and the questions in table 1.1 can open new doorways to delve deeper into curriculum knowledge and skills. Try these questions after a lesson, project, or any significant curriculum experience. Notice how wellness arises from open-hearted reflection and mining for meaning, even if the experience itself is not focused on well-being.

7. *Lifeplay*: Give students a copy of the debrief questions on a card (see p. 263). Invite them to carry this card and use the questions in their lives outside school whenever anything meaningful, challenging or otherwise significant happens. Debrief this lifeplay practice periodically to give students a chance to share and marinate in the experience of mining for meaning throughout their life.

Keywords: card, cognitive, circle, collaborative, emotional, empower, eudaimonia, foundational, gratitude, growth, integration, journal, lifeplay, hedonia, prep-free, social

Taking Refuge: Checking in to Self (Main Move)

Each of us has a safe and nourishing home base. This refuge has no walls, and cannot be seen, yet is eternally available in the *presence of being*. The more purely we can return to this awareness, the more deeply we ground and center ourselves in life. There are several doorways to this home, including watching the breath, feeling the body, or simply listening. Taking refuge (or checking in to self) is a practice of using these doorways to access and expand awareness (being) in the midst of busy lives that tend to be dominated by thinking and doing.

When we are home in this presence, it can feel like a soft, still, awareness of both internal and external experience. Thoughts may still come into this place, but there is a greater capacity to choose whether we get lost in them or add to them. In taking this refuge over and over, key wellness capacities of focus, equanimity, and self-love can be developed. These contribute to greater acceptance of—and flow with—both the outside world and the world within. Naturalist, activist, and writer Terry Tempest Williams understands: "[M]y refuge is not found in my mother, my grandmother, or even the birds of Bear River. My refuge exists in my capacity to love."[28]

Finding and choosing a refuge (foci) that feels stable and grounding for each individual is key. Different people will prefer different refuges as explained in the safety section below. However, once this home base is found, returning to it gently and repeatedly becomes a powerful gift that keeps on giving. The kind-hearted, relaxed awareness cultivated in this practice can gradually seep into the day-to-day interactions of our lives. For example, where technology use can cause addiction, impair social-emotional development, and fracture attention, taking refuge brings concentration, wholeness, and a capacity to connect to self and others.[29]

Just as distraction is grooved through repetition, our loving awareness is also deepened through taking refuge frequently in the ever-available havens of our very own senses, breath, or body. In particular, becoming aware of the inner body (interoception, see p. 22) is a vital sense that will be developed and applied in many activities throughout the book. Remembering to do all this is often the trickiest part, and so this activity offers three natural and effective ways to remember to rediscover our warm home of awareness. While this practice develops multiple well-being domains (see keywords below), it is presented here as a fundamental, foundational practice for all school and life, and it can be introduced by any classroom teacher.

Time is a precious resource for every teacher, and this practice can actually create time. Taking only minutes to explain when woven seamlessly into classroom and life moments, each repetition enables better choices and actions that save time in countless ways. Invite students, and yourself, to take refuge often to discover the profound effect of presence on well-being.

Summary: Create and use different cues to return to presence throughout the day.
Time: 15 minutes (initial), 1–15 seconds (ongoing)
Trust Required: Low

1. *Three Refuges* (1 minute): Invite students to focus on listening, breathing, and feeling in turn. A suggested prompt may be "I will describe three different ways to focus your awareness. For each one, I will invite you to go quiet and see how each one feels, with gentleness, for only a few seconds. It's normal to have thoughts while this happens; see if you can make space for them and not add more." Let them experience each focus below for ten or fifteen seconds, cueing them when to switch. Remind them briefly during each switch that if they forget about the focus to just come back when they can.
   a. *Breathing*: Watching the breath without needing to change it in any way.
   b. *Feeling*: Sensations inside the body, accepting what's there.
   c. *Listening*: To sounds around you, and beyond the room, without judgement.
2. *Returning* (1 minute): Invite students to return to the whole group, gently opening eyes when ready (if they are closed), and noticing what will best support them in returning. This could be some deep breaths, a stretch, yawn, some body movement, rubbing the face, a little self-hug, or whatever feels nourishing.
3. *Choose Refuge* (4 minutes): Ask students what happened during their experience of "taking refuge." They may have had difficulty with one focus, or a more stable grounding with another. Ask them to consider which foci produced more thoughts versus those which felt more immersed and "at home." After a brief discussion, invite students to choose the focus that feels most like a cozy refuge for them personally.

See "Safety" below for more alternatives to breathing, feeling, or listening.
4. *Three Reminders* (4 minutes): Now that students have a focus, invite them to write down responses to the prompts below, giving some thinking time for each. Prompt the group to share a few examples, and make it known that you as teacher are also coming up with ideas and will be participating.
   a. Write down something that happens frequently during the day that you don't think about (e.g., a notification sound, seeing the time, going through a door).
   b. Write a mildly challenging situation that is coming up regularly for you right now.
   c. Write down an obvious or funny change you could make (on your person, at home, in your locker, etc.) that would be hard to miss. For example, switching a bracelet to the opposite wrist, drawing a happy face on your thumb, putting a frog sticker on your phone, or propping a stuffed animal above a bedroom door.
5. *Taking Refuge Lifeplay* (1 minute): Invite everyone (including yourself as teacher) to take the refuge chosen in step 3 whenever any of the reminders in step 4 come up. This could be over a few days or an entire term. It isn't necessary to completely stop whatever is happening to check in, although that may happen as taking refuge typically takes only a few seconds or more. Encourage students to play with the experience, and smile in celebration each time they remember to do it (rather than judging themselves when they do not), for it's a major achievement to *remember* and *return* to loving awareness.
6. *Ongoing Debrief* (5 minutes): Each day for a week, remind the class about the challenge, perhaps sharing a few stories, changes, or insights (see p. 13 for more on debriefing). Emphasize a loving approach where acceptance and equanimity are practiced, rather than a competitive or self-critical stance. Consider having students choose their own name for this practice: grounding, centering, anchoring, taking refuge,

checking in, going quiet, or finding home. Use the practice regularly, and debrief when it feels necessary.
7. *Modeling and Practice* (30 seconds): Model this practice as a teacher by taking refuge yourself during class. For example, take a breath in the middle of a lesson or listen for a moment after a bell rings. Repeat the activity with the whole class as well, perhaps inviting students to lead and/or share their personal check-in process. Eventually, the aim is for a completely self-initiated practice.
8. *Safety*: Trauma or stored emotions may be activated as a person learns to be still and attentive to themselves. Although some release might be beneficial, initial experiences may not be calming, or include over-activation (hyperarousal) or numbness and shutting down (hypoarousal). The following options can help students regulate well.
   a. *Offer choice and flexibility* to help in finding a stable focus or refuge. Use the choices and options available in each activity. Those who feel unsettled focusing on the inner body may find stability in the feet, in one finger, or in keeping their eyes open and simply seeing their surroundings. Taking a few deep breaths might be a helpful refuge for one person, whereas someone living with asthma may find the breath uncomfortable, and instead prefer listening. External foci (seeing the room, listening to sounds) often feel more stable than internal ones (focusing on mental images, auditory thoughts, and inner body feelings).
   b. *Personal agency* must be encouraged, by inviting participants to find and choose what most feels like a stable refuge for them and helps them stay in a relaxed window of calmness. Encourage students to change, blend, or even come up with their own foci—whatever feels most comfortable.
   c. Provide *alternative strategies* and resources, such as self-regulation (see p. 115) or self-compassion (p. 200).

Students living with trauma or other mental health challenges may have external supports they can draw on (see *referral* p. 38).
9. *Integration Strategy*: As taking refuge becomes more automatic, it can be used throughout the school day:
   a. as a transition to bring focus to beginnings and endings of classroom routines;
   b. as a break in the midst of a work or learning session;
   c. as a self-check-in before group or whole class sharing and reflection; and/or
   d. before, during, or after any experience that may be new or challenging.
10. *Schoolwide Extension*: Share this practice with the student body through colleagues or at an assembly. A soft sound played through the public address system can cue everyone—whatever they are doing—to pause for a moment of refuge.

Keywords: card, caring, choice, cognitive, emotional, foundational, integration, lifeplay, mindfulness, prep-free, resilience, safety, schoolwide, short-'n'-safe, spiritual, time-maker

Interoception: Inquiring Within (Main Move)

"Go inside and listen to your body, because your body will never lie to you. Your mind will play tricks, but the way you feel in your heart, in your guts, is the truth."[30]

—Don Miguel Ruiz

See, hear, touch, taste, smell: on the surface, the lesson of the five senses seems as innocent as the young children who learn. There are more than five, but perhaps it's best to keep things simple for young brains. Yet those same brains are constantly receiving sensory signals from the outside world *and* inside the body. The world of sensation doesn't begin on the skin, we can also feel *in*. Yet the five senses all feel *out*, implying that we do not (or cannot) sense the body, and further imprinting society's tendency to avoid feeling what's happening inside us.

But we need to inquire within to be well. Sensing inwardly reveals a rich emotional world, accesses the subtle wisdom of intuition, and provides vital body information we don't get anywhere else.[31] Feeling the inner body (*interoception*) adds a somatic sense to the basic external five, putting us in touch with hunger, heart rate, and breathing, all of which are quite handy for staying alive. A host of other signals are constantly shared in our brains and bodies, mostly without our knowledge. But developing interoception tunes us into a crucial set of signals related to well-being in every domain: our feelings.

Most people have a language for their inner feelings, despite never being taught skills of interoception, or even knowing that it is a sense. Others are numb to their bodies and feelings, especially those living with anxiety, autism, depression, or trauma. Regardless of our inner sensitivity, it's difficult to sort through body sensations, thoughts, and behavior, as each of these are subtle, rapid, and intricately bound up with each other. The good news is that our sense of interoception can be developed. Teachers who immerse themselves in the practice along with students, endorse and reinforce this vital skill.

Whether we are hungry, excited, tense, warm, or elated, interoception is a vital feedback mechanism for physical, cognitive, and emotional well-being.[32] The ability to feel the inner body is associated with self-compassion and emotional regulation, as well as positive body image.[33] Feeling the inner body has benefits for every domain of well-being and so is presented here as a foundational practice of learning and well-being. The various interoception options below need not be done all at once, but explored at different times and in the context of other activities.

> **Summary**: Practice feeling the inner body in different ways.
> **Time**: 5 minutes × 3 (initial), 1–10 seconds (ongoing)
> **Trust Required**: Medium
>
> 1. *Safety*: Students with trauma may have difficulty with interoception, so make any exploration related to the body (and related sharing) invitational and optional. Alternatives to

interoception could be "Taking Refuge" (p. 17). Also remember inner experiences will be unique, so welcome and accept these differences.

2. *Interoception* (3 minutes): Invite students to directly experience interoception in any of the following ways. They will likely need to be told there are more than five senses, with some going inward as well as outward. Thirty seconds is a suggested duration, repeating as desired. Just be sure to practice the skill yourself as a teacher with students.
   a. Invite students to close their eyes to focus on breathing. But not just where the breath leaves the body in the nose or mouth, or on the surface of the chest, also invite them to sense where it is deepest inside the lungs, and how the belly feels.
   b. Invite students to sit quietly and see if they can detect their own heartbeat, without using their fingers to check the pulse. They may close their eyes if it helps. Invite them to locate the feeling in their body, finding the rhythm of their own heart.
   c. Invite students to detect different temperatures, starting on the skin and going deeper, just by sensing. Invite them to place a hand on another part of their body (face, arm, etc.) and notice the contrast, if any, and which is warmer or cooler.

3. *Body Literacy* (5 minutes): Sometimes it can be hard to find words for what we feel. Developing vocabulary for body sensations and feelings can help with relating to them. Try some of the following prompts with students, inviting them to notice and then share three things: *what* happens inside the body, *where* it happens in the body, and any *words* they have for that experience. A basic distinction that can be universally helpful is to notice what feels good (expansion, lightness, warmth) versus what feels bad (contraction, heaviness, coldness).

a. Invite students to notice a particular part of the body, mentally giving a word to the sensation there (hard/soft, stretched/loose, cool/warm) if there is one. Then they stretch that part gently for 30 seconds, and sense again, to note any changes. They then tense the muscles in that part of the body, sense them, relax, sense them again, and so on. Repeat this for rubbed hands, pressing softly or firmly, movements, or other changes such as drinking water or eating something healthy (or junky).
   b. Invite students to think of a happy experience, or something they really love, and notice what happens inside the body, and where, along with the words for it. They may describe warmth, lightness, shivers, expansion in various places inside the body, or use other words—there are no wrong answers.
   c. Invite students to think of a food they dislike, and share their varying inner experience (e.g., tightness in throat, contraction, heaviness in the belly).
   d. Invite students to think of an emotion (or use feels wheels, p. 180) and see if they can sense *where* in the body they feel the emotion and any words to describe it.
4. *Inhabiting Self* (5 minutes): Invite students to spend thirty seconds to a minute getting *inside* each of the following parts of the body. Let them know that the entire continuum of body awareness is okay: from not feeling at all, to a faint sense, to a clear feeling, to a sense of completely *inhabiting* that part. Invite them to feel or even *become* the following:
   a. their hands;
   b. their feet;
   c. the inside of their head, right in the middle of the skull;
   d. their heart, right in the middle of the chest; and/or
   e. the inside of their belly, right in the middle of the abdomen.
5. *Debrief (5 minutes)*: When students begin sharing experiences of interoception and find words to describe inner

feelings, a powerful window to emotional expression and intuition is opened. Use the standard debrief questions (p. 16) and adapt as needed when interoception is used in regular curriculum contexts or with other wellness activities.
6. *Integration Strategy*: Checking into the body can be an intuitive and reliable gauge for preferences (when choosing a learning topic), quality (when deciding if work is completed to a high standard), or to get an initial body sense of where one stands on a complex point of view. See feedback mechanisms (p. 40) for more.
7. *Lifeplay*: Encourage students to continue to access feelings inside their bodies throughout the day, listening to the signals that are available to them. Look for chances to debrief life experiences students may report and how interoception shapes those experiences.

Keywords: card, emotional, foundational, integration, mindfulness, physical, prep-free, resilience

Plumbing the Well: Assessing Well-Being

"The whole purpose of education is to turn mirrors into windows."

—Sydney J. Harris

As teachers embrace well-being outcomes and facilitate learning around well-being, the *assessment* of wellness is a logical next step. Whether well-being is included in formal evaluation or not, assessment can help find gaps, provide feedback for growth, and adjust teaching approaches. Assessment is just as vital for well-being as it is for traditional learning in order to make learning and growth in the various domains of flourishing visible.

This activity provides a set of reflection questions (table 1.2) and a step-by-step process to quickly create well-being assessment tools. Questions are sorted by associated domains to help spotlight particular areas, although the domains are highly interdependent. A starting point is to piggyback a few of these questions onto existing classroom rubrics, tests, or other assessment tools. Teachers can then make their own dedicated well-being assessment tool using the process below or find ready-made online assessments for youth (see p. 31).

Well-being differs from traditional learning in that it is cultivated socially, and includes teachers in the learning. For these reasons, in planning for balanced well-being assessment, consider using the following:

- mostly diagnostic and formative approaches (before and during learning respectively);
- primarily self-assessment, with minimal peer or teacher assessment only if trust is deep;
- observations and conversations, in addition to self-reflection; and/or
- teacher self-reflection to guide personal educator wellness, rather than being in the typical role as an assessor of students.

Summary: Create a variety of valid, relevant assessment tools that gauge well-being.
Time: Varies
Trust Required: Low

1. *Prep*: Create a well-being assessment tool using table 1.2 and the process below.
   a. Consider the time span for the assessment, which could range from a single activity of a few minutes to a period of several weeks or more. This determines the prompt that precedes the questions you select below. Some examples follow:
      i. "To what degree *did today's activity* contribute to the following items . . ."
      ii. "To what degree do you agree with each item below, based on how you have felt *over the past learning unit of three weeks* . . ."
   b. Select one or more questions from table 1.2 to include in the assessment tool. Fewer questions are recommended,

as well-being domains are rich, and asking for reflection in many areas at once may be counterproductive. Also choose a response scale, which could be as simple as "true or false," or more nuanced with a four-to-seven point scale including "strongly disagree, disagree, somewhat disagree, neutral, somewhat agree, agree, or strongly agree."
c. Choose how to administer your assessment tool, using a balanced variety of assessment strategies. For example, the assessment tool could be used as
   i. a personal self-reflection, completed individually;
   ii. a prompt sheet for partner talk, teacher interview, or group conversation; and/or
   iii. an observation scale to note well-being skills or behaviors in action.
d. Add a space at the bottom of your tool for open self-reflection or comments, whether written or drawn out in conversation. Comments could include the following:
   i. self-reflective feedback to improve well-being;
   ii. personal challenges to well-being, and resources or support needed;
   iii. personal changes in well-being over time, and their impact; and/or
   iv. general thoughts, feelings or connections made.
2. *Assess* (time varies): Distribute the assessment tool to students, preferably at the outset of learning to build understanding of well-being criteria in different domains. Also give students time during well-being activities to check into the assessment, and consider if any positive changes have occurred, or what they might do differently. The assessments could theoretically be collected, but they are best left with students for personal reflection over time. The possibilities are endless: keep it light, fun, and positive. A growth mindset is key, since the purpose of assessment is to improve well-being (er, and learning).
3. *Safety*: Assessments of well-being ought to *contribute* to wellness, so *self-assessment* is recommended, especially where group trust has not yet been firmly established. Encourage

honesty and self-compassionate in self-assessment, including for the teacher.
4. *Integration Strategy*: Teachers with less time to assess wellness in a standalone way can insert these questions into existing classroom tools and tasks.

Keywords: cognitive, choice, emotional, environmental, eudaimonia, foundational, get-to-know, hedonia, integration, physical, resilience, safety, social, spiritual, support

Table 1.2. Well-Being Self-Assessment Reflection Questions

Domain	Reflection Question
Cognitive	I am engaged and interested in my life, with diverse hobbies and interests.
Cognitive	I become so absorbed, sometimes time passes without noticing.
Cognitive	I feel aware of what's happening around me and inside me.
Cognitive	I feel calm and composed about what happens in life, good or bad.
Cognitive	I have creativity, intellect, and a good intuition.
Cognitive	I'm a good decision maker and problem solver.
Cognitive	I have a healthy relationship toward my thoughts.
Cognitive	In general, I feel cognitively well.
Emotional	I have words to describe my feelings, and I express them.
Emotional	I feel grateful most of the time, for most things.
Emotional	I usually don't feel anxious, angry, or sad.
Emotional	I've been feeling cheerful or joyful.
Emotional	I have a good sense of how others are feeling.
Emotional	I can influence and manage my emotions when I need to.
Emotional	My feelings are a rich and useful part of my life.
Emotional	In general, I feel emotionally well.
Environmental	I enjoy spending time in natural spaces, even remote ones.
Environmental	I value and protect the environment and take action to protect it.
Environmental	In general, I feel connected and nourished to all life and the earth.
Eudaimonic	I know who I really am and live in alignment with my true self.
Eudaimonic	I have found my purpose in life: life is valuable and interesting.
Eudaimonic	I feel engaged in school and other responsibilities.
Eudaimonic	I am making progress toward meaningful goals.
Eudaimonic	I feel like I am excelling at something worthwhile (or on the way).
Eudaimonic	I contribute to the well-being of others.
Eudaimonic	My life aligns with my strengths, passions, and values.
Eudaimonic	In general, I feel like I live a meaningful, authentic life.

(continued)

Table 1.2. (continued)	
Domain	Reflection Question
Physical	I regularly eat a balance of protein, whole grains, veggies, and fruit.
Physical	I regularly get 150 minutes of hard-breathing activity each week.
Physical	I feel like my sleep habits keep me refreshed and healthy.
Physical	I rarely or never use alcohol/drugs, cut myself, or binge.
Physical	If I have sex, I use protection and respect my partner.
Physical	I take care of my health and hygiene, and I get health care when needed.
Physical	In general, I feel physically well.
Resilience	I accept what happens, without too much judgment.
Resilience	I feel good about my capabilities and have self-compassion and self-love.
Resilience	I feel optimistic, yet realistic.
Resilience	I tend to focus on what I can change rather than stuff outside my control.
Resilience	I welcome uncertainty or challenge as a vital part of life.
Resilience	I'm able to experience difficult things without avoiding or numbing.
Resilience	I'm strong and flexible in the face of adversity.
Resilience	Setbacks or adversity typically result in some kind of growth for me.
Resilience	In general, I'm able to deal with adversity well.
Safety	I have a stable place to live where I feel safe, free, and have basic needs met.
Safety	I feel safe in the classroom, physically, socially, and emotionally.
Social	I can manage conflict well, whether it involves me or others.
Social	I feel deeply close to somebody.
Social	I feel empathy and understanding for others.
Social	I feel like I belong.
Social	I feel like I have good relationships with family, friends, or others.
Social	I feel loved.
Social	I reach out for and accept help or support from others when I need it.
Social	In general, I feel socially connected.
Spiritual	I have experiences that take me beyond the norm or myself in some way.
Spiritual	I feel a deep connection with something to the point of being one with it.
Spiritual	I feel joy, peace, or awe for some parts of this life, or a life beyond.
Spiritual	In general, I feel spiritually well.

SUPPLEMENTARIES: SHORT, SIMPLE, SAFE, OR SEARCHABLE WELL-BEING

- *Announcing Well-Being* is the public broadcasting of wellness tips during school announcements, and on the school website or social media platforms to extend well-being widely. Announcing every day may be intrusive, so consider one-week blitzes or one day a week (Wellness Wednesdays are a classic). Consider switching themes monthly using the domains of well-being. *Search terms*: wellness, tips, announcements.
- *Virtues Vocab* enlarges student understanding of character strengths and virtues (such as integrity, kindness and humility), which have been determined to be universal and good for humanity.[34] Students can choose a virtue to research and share with the class or use online lists to support exploring virtues in the context of any activity. Free posters, cards or definitions can also be downloaded from a variety of sites, particularly the VIA Character Institute, which also has a youth survey.[35] *Search terms*: universal, virtues, list.
- *Well Seated* encourages teachers to choose and use a variety of seating arrangements depending on the needs and input of students. Grids, pairs, quads, pods, horseshoes, rows, corners, and circles offer freshness and wellness, especially when combined with random, visible groupings (see p. 84). Students quickly get used to setting up various configurations, including a home option. *Search terms*: classroom, seating, arrangements.
- *Well-being Assessments* found online from educational organizations can spark discussions about any domain of well-being, and augment teacher-created materials (see p. 26). *Search terms*: well-being, assessment, tool, youth, student, [domain].

❷

SAFETY

Essential Needs and Freedoms

"I've learned that people will forget what you said, people will forget what you did, but people will never forget how you made them feel."

—Maya Angelou

Safety is the foundational pillar of well-being, since most everything well and good in the classroom depends on it—achievement, attendance, curiosity, and more. While there's no such thing as an absolutely safe classroom, *safer* classrooms are definitely within reach. Teachers have a powerful influence in creating spaces where both students and staff feel

- safer physically (free from harm);
- safer emotionally (free from abuse and oppression); and
- a sense of agency (the autonomy to make choices in life).

Making this difference matters for every student, but it matters even more for those who have had their essential needs or freedoms violated. One half of adolescents will have had an adverse childhood experience (traumatic event) such as abuse, neglect, or separation. Teens who identify as Black, Indigenous, and/or 2SLGBTQ+ have significantly more. One in ten students will have had three or more.[1] These events have lasting, negative impacts on well-being, as do systemic oppressions such as racism, homophobia, or poverty.

Reagan, sixteen years old, wants to get into a skilled trade but has been to three schools after several suspensions for fighting and swearing. These incidents occurred while her mother was in an addiction treatment center, and she was forced to move in with her estranged father. Her father subjected her to verbal and emotional abuse, and he could not provide adequate food or clothing.

Fortunately for Reagan, her manufacturing teacher (who had grown up in poverty) took the time to earn her trust, find out what was happening, and get help. Reagan was provided with foster care, and she is progressing on a pathway to apprentice as a machinist.

While teachers can't choose what students bring to class, they can learn to meet them with empathy and understanding. Being a pedagogue or a content expert is great, but any learning requires these key safety essentials:

- a safe, loving classroom environment (what teachers do);
- open lines of communication (what teachers say); and
- personal qualities that enhance safety (who teachers are).

These essentials involve balancing expectations with support, sharing power, and giving students voice and choice. Whether with racism, poverty, or any form of trauma, eliminating individual, school and systemic barriers requires an active, rather than passive, approach.

Ibram Kendi explains that being "non-racist" isn't enough: "What's the problem with being 'not racist'? It is a claim that signifies neutrality: 'I am not a racist, but neither am I aggressively against racism.' But there is no neutrality in the racism struggle. The opposite of 'racist' isn't 'not racist.' It is 'antiracist.'"[2] While some teachers may have little or no experience with anti-oppression, or providing the essentials of safety, it is a moral imperative for them to learn to do so. This means acknowledging systems and situations that negatively impact particular students or groups, and taking on their ethical and professional duty to address them. Clearly committing to this stance publicly in the classroom creates openings for students to express their lived experiences.

This chapter addresses safety essentials, creating a foundation for journeying into other wellness domains. Every domain helps, with the cognitive, emotional, resilience, and social domains contributing significantly to safety. While it's impossible to create perfect safety before engaging in any learning or well-being, having a base bodes well for the journey.

QUALITIES OF SAFER HUMAN BEINGS

Words that convey a commitment to safety are important. Positive, proactive *actions* to make a classroom safer speak louder than any words. But the *way* a teacher interacts with their students speaks louder than any words or actions. A stable, caring, and responsive teacher presence or being inspires a corresponding peace and warmheartedness in students, all of which adds layers of safety to the classroom community.

For these reasons, the following qualities are a focus of the various chapter activities throughout the book and are intended for both students and teachers. Teachers who see these pursuits as being for students as much as themselves can create beautiful, harmonious classroom communities. Reference the keywords (see appendix, p. 261) to focus on particular qualities.

- *Aware* people notice what influences well-being in themselves and others; they then choose healthy, skillful decisions and actions (keyword *mindfulness*).
- *Compassionate* people inspire caring classrooms, especially when they are also kind to themselves in balance. Personal and community wellness thrive as one (keyword *caring*).
- *Connected* people build healthy relationships and contribute to prosocial classroom activities, in balance with independent work (keyword *social*).

- *Flexible* people adapt, find alternatives, and flow with classroom life. They reflect the fluidity of learning and value student choices (keywords *choice, resilience*).
- *Grateful* people imbue school life and everyone around them with a precious and rare commodity: thankfulness and appreciation for what's going well (keyword *gratitude*).
- *Joyful* people are simply delightful: their positive radiance streams outward and warms others in all directions, since happiness is contagious (keyword *hedonia*).
- *Peaceful* people cultivate inner calm and exude that tranquility such that it can be felt by all present (keyword *mindfulness*).
- *Responsive* people take action reliably in the face of student needs. They follow through with issues in a restorative way to relieve tension and build safer communities, reassuring everyone in the process (keywords *restorative*).
- *Vulnerable* people share deeply and show their authentic selves. They admit when they don't know, acknowledge harm caused, share power, and let their humanity be seen. Their vulnerability validates emotional expression and wellness (keyword *emotional*).

Making the Invisible Visible

Even if a teacher somehow possessed all these wondrous qualities and did everything possible to make the classroom safer, students will still feel their own subjective sense of safety. This felt sense changes constantly, and it is often left unspoken. In addition, it can be difficult for students to share their feelings of security, due to social conditioning not to emote, or from a lack of role models for emotional expression. Social media superficiality doesn't help. It's telling that "too much information (TMI)," "oversharing," or even "vulnerability hangover" are commonly heard, but never "too little information" or "undersharing." Making feelings visible is key.

For these reasons, authentic student feedback is necessary to guide safety efforts (just as ongoing assessment guides teaching and learning). This feedback comes from building relationships, soliciting anonymous communication, and learning about the lives of students, rather than making assumptions. Teachers who are aware of their own privilege (for example the advantages of being white, straight, or cisgender), and/

or power (for example the positional power of being a teacher) are less likely to make unfounded assumptions about students or their safety. With honest feedback, it is possible to detect and disrupt power dynamics or larger systems of oppression (like sexism, racism, or homophobia) that play out in a classroom.

The implications of all this for teachers is to maintain healthy lines of communication by consistently encouraging openness, whenever and however it arises in class. The feedback and monitoring strategies in this chapter (see p. 40) provide ways to do this: assessing trust, informing next steps, and opening up communication to develop wellness in a safer way.

Levels of Trust Required

Over time, by using the approaches provided in this and other domains, a depth of classroom assurance may open the door for activities requiring deeper trust. To guide in this deepening, all activities have an associated level of *trust required* as follows:

- *Low:* the activity is safer to use with groups just getting to know each other, and/or groups that have not yet developed significant degrees of trust or safety.
- *Medium:* the activity is safer for groups who have built some community trust over time.
- *High:* the activity is safer where there is a significant degree of courage and trust, likely built over an extended period of time working on well-being and safety together.

Teachers considering these levels will seek student feedback and check their own personal feelings of safety in order to choose activities that match classroom trust.

For this reason, perhaps the most important person whose feelings must be considered by the teacher is . . . the teacher. As the adult in the room, their capacity to hold space is vital. This requires teachers to notice their own feelings, grow personal traits, work with discomfort, and seek support when needed. This is especially true since well-being activities invite teachers to participate authentically as well as facilitate—a delicate but life-affirming experience.

In doing so, teachers can care deeply while not feeling responsible for the totality of their students' lives. They may also share personally when such sharing benefits students. After handing back a test that many of his grade 9 students bombed, Mr. Fochler shared his own experience of failure in school and in trying to become a licensed pilot. This led to a discussion of factors that contribute to success and how Mr. Fochler could help get students back on track. Safer spaces may feel comfortable, but healthy conversations will require groups to move in and out of comfort zones on the pathway to well-being.

Indeed, critical conversations around well-being and equity will require discomfort. Teachers who welcome discomfort, participate fully, share openly, and grow with students can inspire great trust and safety. Teachers with lived experience (or at least some knowledge) of an oppressed group add extra layers of trust. Teachers who cannot acknowledge their gaps and implicit biases (such as ableism or white supremacy) whether from ignorance or shame, put safety at risk and shut down conversations. But when teachers are aware of social position, power, and seek ongoing feedback, high trust activities become accessible and safety flourishes.

Lyn had a lovely grade 7 class with students who seemed more than willing to share in classroom discussions. Devi in particular was sunny and vocal, but Lyn noticed her face scrunch up whenever Elisa or Amanda said anything. Lyn didn't make much of it but continued to build relationships. It wasn't until Devi made a nasty comment, which seemed to come from nowhere, that Lyn asked to speak to her after class. Devi was sullen and silent, but she eventually shared that the girls had bullied her in grade 6 about her accent, and nobody did anything. Lyn decided to offer a restorative process with all the girls and to seek administrative support.

When to Get Help

Teachers like Lyn who take time to build relationships can uncover all kinds of information that could help create a safer space. But it's also critical to recognize when to refer students to school administration, counselors, external agencies, or all three. While wellness practices are wonderful and commonplace, students in crisis need additional sup-

SAFETY

port. In some cases reporting is required by law. The indicators below can help identify those in need, but they are not exhaustive. Therefore, teachers must err on the side of caution when there are warning signs, or they feel out of their depth, and refer students for support who:

- disclose suicidal ideation;
- have signs of self-harm such as burns or cuts, or disclose a desire to self-harm;
- need, or seems to need, protection from abuse or neglect;
- pose any danger to their own well-being or that of others;
- explicitly ask for help or counseling;
- have troubling content in written work or in what they say;
- seem to be struggling in dealing with a personal situation, trauma, or loss;
- are overly aggressive, anxious, apathetic, confused, dependent, depressed, or withdrawn;
- have multiple absences, significant missed work, or want to drop out of school;
- show marked changes in appearance, hygiene, or behavior; and/or
- disclose or indicate any significant sign of well-being or academic vulnerability.

Teachers do well to proactively familiarize themselves with the referral pathway for students of concern as well as available support or resources before issues arise. Whether or not students get help beyond the classroom, the teacher remains a crucial part of their ongoing wellness. The activities in this book are designed to benefit all but can be vital for some who require additional care. Where possible, seek the guidance and support of school-based professional staff, and/or external staff and agencies, in any well-being efforts.

Key Messages

- An anti-oppressive stance makes classrooms safer for learning and well-being.

- A safe space, open communication (including anonymous feedback), and positive human qualities help build a safety foundation, in addition to the activities in this chapter.
- Safety and community deepen with every other wellness domain, allowing higher trust activities to be used, based on the "trust required" provided with each activity.
- Teacher participation in wellness activities alongside students helps validate the practices, as well as build more safety and classroom trust.
- Refer students for external support when needed.

SAFETY ACTIVITIES

Anonymous Feedback Channels (Main Move)

"No news is good news" is actually bad news in the classroom. It's vital for teachers to know what students are thinking and feeling to create a safer learning environment. Whether after a learning task, wellness activity, or any classroom experience, it's important to seek feedback and minimize the risk for youth to give it authentically. Anonymous feedback channels do just that, helping students surface how they really feel to create courageous spaces.

Getting authentic student feedback using the four options below reduces harm and saves time that can be wasted on unproductive or unsafe classroom activity. As feedback is gathered in these ways, confidentiality must be preserved by not revealing comments that could be attributed (or assumed to be attributed) to particular students. The teacher need not know or reveal the source of any feedback, what is required is to respond in general ways that address concerns. Some example feedback and possible teacher follow-up actions are shown in table 2.1.

Getting students to share can be risky for them, and they will likely not know *how* to make things safer. Therefore, after getting any such feedback, it's critical for teachers to review it and report back to students. Failing to respond promptly erodes trust, no matter how much feedback is sought. Following up on feedback with visible actions that boost safety lets students know the teacher has their best interests at heart, fostering deep trust and even deeper well-being.

Table 2.1. Sample Anonymous Feedback and Teacher Responses

Example Student Feedback	Teacher Followup Suggestions
"People think that everyone brown is either Sikh or Muslim; it's so frustrating."	Tell students you have heard their feedback and are taking action, without sharing this particular comment. Do some personal learning as a teacher to know your students' history, heritage, language, and religion, providing ways to affirm identities and connect with students. Invite community members or caregivers into the classroom, making curriculum connections where possible. Represent diverse identities in lesson materials, and lead discussions to surface and dispel biases and misconceptions about a broad range of identities, without spotlighting a particular group.
"I didn't like sharing with the whole class."	Tell students you have heard their feedback and are taking action. Ensure "right to pass" is a universal agreement, congratulate students who pass, and model passing as a teacher, to boost safety for others. Provide more options in activities for personal reflection, partner, or whole group sharing.
"When you raise your voice to ask us to simmer down, it sometimes feels intense."	Tell students you have heard their feedback and are taking action. Acknowledge that you have been frustrated, raised your voice, and that impacted on the class. Apologize, and commit to take extra care to respond more gently in future. Ask for student feedback on this particular issue again in a week or two to see if feelings have changed.
[Student scores "zero" for safety in the context of a whole class circle activity.]	Tell students you have heard their feedback and will stop doing whole class circle activities. Consider the safety considerations for circles (see p. 61) and take actions to increase student safety, or switch to different approaches until the feedback changes.
[One or two students in the class feel unsafe, but don't say why.]	Tell students you have heard their feedback and are taking action. Consider any prior events that may be impacting the situation. Continue with student relationship-building and 1:1 interviews to potentially surface and address concerns, ensuring privacy and confidentiality is preserved.
[A significant number of students feel unsafe in different ways.]	Tell students you have heard their feedback and are taking action. Choose some or all of the following options to build individual safety, and seek their feedback regularly on them: • Use lower risk activities in general. • Use more individual and self-reflective activities. • Use activities from the safety, social, emotional, and resilience domains.

As students indicate higher levels of safety, more challenging activities can be introduced as per the levels of trust (p. 37). Choosing trust-appropriate activities engages students optimally and develops qualities of safer human beings (p. 35), particularly vulnerability. This does not mean vulnerability in the sense of being easily hurt but as a strength. Researcher and storyteller Brené Brown explains: "The definition of vulnerability is uncertainty, risk, and emotional exposure. Vulnerability is not weakness; it's our most accurate measure of courage. When the barrier to vulnerability is about safety, the question becomes: are we willing to create courageous spaces so we can be fully seen?"[3]

> **Summary**: Seek anonymous feedback in different ways frequently throughout learning.
> **Time**: Varies
> **Trust Required**: Low
>
> 1. *Exit Passes* (2 minutes) are paper slips given out before the end of class that students complete and drop off when they exit (e.g., in a box by the door). Focus on one or two specific activities for which feedback is being sought, rather than just saying "today's class." Tell students the passes are anonymous and confidential. Sample prompts follow:
>   a. How safe did you feel during the microlab activity today, from 0 (not at all) to 5 (completely safe)? If applicable, what could help you feel safer?
>   b. Check out next week's activity [linked] where we will sketch a line representing your life's ups and downs. How safe might you feel doing this sharing:
>   i. with nobody, just reflecting privately (0 to 5)?
>   ii. with a single partner (0 to 5)?
>   iii. with the whole class, but only if you wish to (0 to 5)?
>   iv. What might help make this activity safer for you?
> 2. *Snowballs* (2 minutes) are crumpled up papers on which students can write anonymous questions or concerns. These get tossed into a bowl or box in the center of a circle (who doesn't want to throw snowballs in class?) The teacher then has options:

a. Collect the box, read the comments outside of class, and report back promptly. Safety is created only when students know their concerns are being read *and* effective follow-up actions are being taken within a short time frame.
b. Read a random snowball to themselves, and then choose to:
    i. read it aloud to the class, or give to a student to read;
    ii. invite whole class discussion;
    iii. respond immediately, or in the near future, with follow-up actions;
    iv. save the snowball to address privately and follow up later.
3. *1:1 Check-Ins* are short, private, interviews held between student and teacher, ensuring that each student is interviewed over time. Conduct the interviews in a quiet corner or hallway. Assure students their feedback won't affect grades in any way. Talk about previous feedback or ongoing classroom activity to give students something to talk about. Then get into how students are feeling about the class and what might make things feel even better.
4. *Online Surveys/Chats* can be used in place of any of the above. The search terms *anonymous classroom poll survey* will give free, web-based options that do not require a student log in or share personal information.
5. *Debrief*: Class discussions will not likely feel safer than anonymous feedback, but may be used to ask for student input around how to get feedback. Inviting a colleague, school counselor, or administrator to gather feedback on the teacher's behalf may help some students open up and be more forthcoming.
6. *Integration Strategy*: Use anonymous feedback in conjunction with almost *any* learning experience to get feedback on curriculum, resources, learning tasks, lessons, assessment, classroom routines, and more. When teachers find a channel that works for them and is comfortable for students, it can be

used repeatedly for ongoing program feedback. As always, balance gathering feedback with reporting back and following up to raise trust.
7. *Schoolwide Extension*: Schools and districts typically conduct anonymous student surveys around student safety. If your district has a research department, they may be able to help design effective instruments at the school level, or board data will be available by school to provide ready-made feedback. It is important to get feedback at times other than the end of the year, and publicly follow up with students so that they know their feedback is being heard and acted upon.
8. *Safety*: With anonymous feedback, students may disclose signs of distress (see p. 39). Teachers must share this information with administration or support staff for follow up, even if the feedback was anonymous.

Keywords: caring, empower, foundational, integration, safety, schoolwide, short-'n'-safe, support, time-maker

Classroom Agreements (Main Move)

Creating and upholding community agreements with students shares power and sets the stage for shared responsibility, accountability, peace, and well-being. This activity is best done after some basic relationships have been established, so perhaps not on the first day. The most important phase of the activity is during the rest of the year, in monitoring, upholding, and maintaining the agreements. As a fundamental and ongoing practice of community building, agreements will save more time than will ever be spent on them, by proactively avoiding issues and creating classroom harmony.

The democracy and relationships developed in creating the agreements must continue beyond the initial creation into the ongoing monitoring and maintenance phase. It is essential to refer to agreements

SAFETY

regularly, and hold everyone in the classroom community, including staff, accountable to them in order for the process to have integrity. Agreements are not just about making a chart paper together, but co-creating a space for student voice, agency, and safety.

> **Summary**: Students and teachers create and uphold classroom agreements.
> **Time**: 30 minutes (initial), 1–10 minutes (ongoing)
> **Trust Required**: Low
>
> 1. *Prep* (2 minutes): Gather markers, scrap paper and chart paper.
> 2. *Initial Creation* (30 minutes)
>   a. *Introduce* (1 minute): Model the qualities you hope for in the classroom, such as peace or authenticity, with an opening statement that comes from the heart. Talk about your intentions and what is important to you, such as creating a safe space for everyone's success. Take an anti-oppressive stance by conveying a willingness to confront and challenge bias and bullying. This gives students permission to share more openly, instead of saying what they think the teacher wants to hear.
>   b. *Barriers* (10 minutes): Students are given a sticky note (or scrap paper) to brainstorm one thing that *gets in the way of* them being or doing their best in class. Limiting to one thing forces a consideration of what is most important. These are crumpled up and placed outside the circle. The teacher opens and reads them one by one, writing them in the outside circle, combining where appropriate. Rewriting preserves anonymity, which may be important at this delicate stage.
>   c. *Supports* (10 minutes): Repeat step 2b except that students write one thing that *supports* them being and doing their best. These are placed inside the circle.
>   d. *Group Discussion* (5 minutes): Edits are made to any agreement, inside or outside the circle, by the whole

group. The teacher may add anything vital that's still missing, such as disrespectful language or right to pass. Doing this is rarely necessary, since the group will likely create a fairly complete set, and these can be modified throughout the year in any case.

   e. *Signing and Posting* (4 minutes): The teacher asks if everyone agrees to the agreements and can commit to follow them. Further discussion can be held, if needed, to reach consensus. Everyone then signs the paper, which is posted in the room. Teachers may photograph, print, and mount the agreements in a frame for hanging or distribute signed copies to each student (though they may change).

3. *Monitoring* (ongoing): Throughout the school year, students and teachers can point out when they feel behavior is "outside the circle" of the agreements. For milder transgressions, teachers simply address students directly and ask for a change. Some policies, such as discriminatory language protocols, may be the teacher's responsibility alone to notice and address. Responding with compassion and firmness to disrespectful behavior is a vital opportunity to create safety. So too is teacher vulnerability to describe the impact on themselves (not just the student or students who caused harm, or those impacted). Students and teachers may collectively decide how to address violations. In more serious breaches, restorative practices may be employed (see p. 133).

4. *Shining* (ongoing): Teachers and students watch for, and point out, positive efforts made "inside the circle" to increase goodwill. Recognizing and celebrating when agreements are upheld, or protected, is a nourishing and positive aspect of the process, which may otherwise feel like a bunch of rules. A classroom with a shining inner circle is a beautiful thing to behold and place to learn.

5. *Maintenance* (periodic, 5 minutes): Schedule time during the term to review the agreements. A short, private, anonymous assessment could be conducted to get honest feedback about

whether the class is living up to the agreements. Follow up with a discussion of any necessary changes in the agreements or the monitoring. Maintenance can also occur spontaneously if the community feels strongly that change is needed.
6. *Debrief* (optional): Debriefing thoughts and feelings about the agreements, particularly to draw out the *impact* on students. Make relevant connections to other areas of life where agreements are made (or broken), including the teacher's own classroom experiences as a student.
7. *Safety*: The teacher must be willing and able to keep the integrity of the agreements through effective follow-up for errant behavior. Students may become more involved in this process, but only after a significant degree of trust has been built in the classroom.

Keywords: caring, collaborative, choice, get-to-know, emotional, empower, eudaimonia, foundational, icebreaker, restorative, safety, social, space

A Loving Container: Making the Classroom a Home

"It matters that students feel safe, it matters that students feel calm."[4]

—Daniel Goleman

Teachers don't get to design their classrooms from scratch, let alone have a consistent room in grades 7–12. However, consulting with students on a few changes goes a long way to cultivating safety. The checklist below captures research-based approaches to create comfortable, calming, flexible, and safer classrooms.[5]

Take some time to survey your own space, visit other classrooms, talk to colleagues, and assign a priority to various checklist items:

- immediately helpful/do-able (do now and check off);
- worthwhile at some point (put a "?" or note to do later); or
- unworkable (strike through and move on).

While some items may be out of reach for some classrooms, all are reasonable, and even small changes can go a long way. If a window won't open, can a plant be added? If the furniture can't be replaced, can one item be swapped? If a human rights speaker isn't available, can posters be displayed representing global perspectives? Keep in mind that comfort for one may be chaos to another. Seek student feedback in the process of creating a loving container.

> **Summary**: Make physical changes to create a calmer, safer, more beautiful classroom space.
> **Time**: Varies
> **Trust Required**: Low
>
> - *Fixes*: Request repairs for climate control, lighting, tiles, windows, drapes, or other basics. A quiet, well-lit, comfortable environment with good air circulation contributes significantly to achievement, comfort, and safety.
> - *Flexible Furniture*: Swap out attached desks and chairs for separated versions, and replace giant group-sized desks with smaller (and more flexible) desks where possible. Add caps to chair legs or wheels to whiteboards to quiet and ease movement respectively. See *Well Seated* (p. 31) for more on flexible classroom configurations.
> - *Alternative Furniture*: Replace or augment furniture with alternatives, such as (in order of most affordable/convenient first) cushions, yoga mats, yoga balls, standing desks, bean-bag chairs, mobile seating, adjustable chairs, wobbly chairs, or rocking chairs. Replacing everything is not necessary or desirable because flexibility is key. Supplement rather than replace if there is space in a corner or at the back.
> - *Defront*: Move the teacher's desk to the side or remove it altogether.
> - *Walls*: Showcase student work, art, and/or photos of pets and families, perhaps in empty frames for a touch of class. En-

sure everyone is represented. Consider having a feature wall with other walls empty, neutral or in soothing, warm colors to avoid clutter and leave at least 25 percent neutral, blank wall space.[6] Students can use this space to create and/or post learning resources as needed. Do not post grades publicly.
- *Inspiration*: Post and discuss well-being quotations, photos of inspiring role models, short stories, or other inspiration on an ongoing basis. Students may select most or all of these items. Be sure to avoid stereotypes in the representation, for example by representing Black identity only through entertainment or sports.
- *Light*: Let in natural light where possible, and consider balancing the time with lights bright versus having one row of lights off (without making it dark). In the latter case, consider adding a warm table lamp or string of lights.
- *Sight*: Project a forest, ocean fishes, or other soothing scene on a screen *sometimes*.
- *Sound*: Play soothing instrumental music or natural, background sounds *sometimes*.
- *Sense:* Provide fidget toys such as pipe cleaners or small plushies on student desks or in a break box (p. 52). Resistance bands tied between desk legs can serve as a foot rest/fidget tamer.
- *Comfy Corner:* Create a safe zone with a comfy chair, light, and soothing objects.
- *Spaces:* Create areas (where possible) that allow for collaboration or reference.
- *Tools:* Provide extra writing implements, paper, personal whiteboards, or other materials for students who may forget them, or never get them from home.

Keywords: caring, choice, foundational, physical, safety, space

Making the Invisible Visible: Semi-Anonymous Feedback

The semi-anonymous feedback channels offered in table 2.2 provide several ways to get a rapid sense of how students are doing, helping make invisible feelings more visible. Teachers can choose one or more approaches, or give students a voice in which they prefer.

Augment these methods with the fully anonymous feedback channels (see p. 40) to get a more complete picture of safety. Seeking feedback, acknowledging when it is received, and responding to it decisively and compassionately is vital for safer classrooms.

Table 2.2. Semi-Anonymous Feedback Channels

Methods	Signals	Learning Context	Feeling Context	Note
Thumbs	up	"I get it"	"I'm good"	Thumbs can be held high or kept more private by hiding them in front of the body.
	sideways	"Not sure"	"Meh"	
	down	"I'm lost"	"I'm not OK"	
Fist to Five	5 fingers	"I can teach it"	"I love this"	Can also be used for consensus testing or decision making.
	4 fingers	"I get it totally"	"I'm good with this"	
	3 fingers	"I get it, mostly"	"I can live with this"	
	2 fingers	"I get part of it"	"Minor issues"	
	1 finger	"I need help"	"Major issues"	
	0 fingers (fist)	"I'm lost"	"No way"	
Cards	green card	"I get it"	"I'm good"	Cards can be left out on desks during work time to signal whether support is needed.
	yellow card	"Not sure"	"Meh"	
	red card	"I'm lost"	"I'm not OK"	
Interoception	[expansion]	"I get it"	"I'm good"	See p. 22 for details on interoception.
	neutral	"Not sure"	"Meh"	
	[contraction]	"I'm lost"	"I'm not OK"	

Summary: Use signals to get quick, non-verbal feedback on how students are doing.
Time: 10 seconds
Trust Required: Low

1. *Prep*: Create sets of red, yellow, and green cards on mini keyrings (optional).
2. *Explain* (2 minutes): Explain and practice one of the methods from table 2.2 with students in the context of a lesson. Tell students they can make their vote more or less public by holding it high or keeping it in front of the body. Note that these methods complement, not replace, completely anonymous feedback channels (p. 40).
3. *Test* (10 seconds): Use the method a few times in the same class, for example,
    a. "Do you feel ready to try this now that I've explained it?" (before)
    b. "How comfortable do you feel right now?" (during)
    c. Does anyone feel confused at this point? (during)
    d. "How did everyone feel about the thumball activity?" (after)
    e. Tell me honestly, how cool was that? (after)
    f. How are you feeling? (any time)
4. *Integration Strategy*: These mechanisms originated in support of learning and curriculum, so they are naturally effective in that context. Seek feedback before, during, and after any learning cycle, whether a single step in a lesson, a single activity, or an entire unit.
5. *Safety*: In some groups certain hand signals may have offensive meanings or no meaning. This can be acknowledged by emphasizing a positive intention or using an alternative. While there are no perfectly universal body gestures or facial expressions across different cultures, there are common expressions for many emotions (see p. 182).

Keywords: caring, empower, foundational, integration, safety, schoolwide, short-'n'-safe, support, time-maker

SUPPLEMENTARIES: SHORT, SIMPLE, OR SEARCHABLE SAFETY

- *Break Boxes* are left out in the classroom for students who need a break or used at the teacher's discretion.[7] The box could include pipe cleaners, squishy balls, modeling clay/putty, (weighted) plush toys, mindful coloring books, puzzle books (illusion, hidden object), fidget toys, origami, and worry stones.
- *Call Me by My True Name* recognizes that mispronouncing (or avoiding) student names are microaggressions that have a lasting negative impact.[8] Make the first page of your class list a phonetic pronunciation column and use it. If you aren't sure, ask a student privately to teach you to say their name perfectly, write down the phonetics, and practice until they confirm you've got it right. *Search terms*: pronounce, student, names.
- *Content Warnings* give notice about upcoming content that might have a negative impact, particularly for those with trauma. Such material could relate to abuse of any kind (including abusive language), hate speech/acts, mental disorders or illness, self-harm, systems of oppression, violence, death, grief, or war. Before using a warning, consider if there's another way to address the learning that doesn't elevate risk. If giving a content warning, do it ahead of time to give students options about whether and how to engage with the content, and to seek support. Some examples follow:
    - "Next week we are going to watch a video of a dissection of a frog. This might trigger unwelcome or distressing thoughts for some. Students may ask for or seek support, discuss concerns or accommodations with a teacher or counselor, or request an alternative lesson."
    - "Next week the class will be learning about reactions to stressful events such as freeze, fight, or flight, with the intention of becoming more aware of such events and typical reactions. Students may ask for or seek support, discuss concerns or accomodations with a teacher or counselor, or request an alternative lesson."
- *Go Slow to Go Fast* is the wisdom of using the first days of school for community building, quiet breaks, and well-being activities, along with some simple and predictable curricular routines. By

forming relationships and building wellness early on, students will be able to learn effectively and efficiently all year long, and problems are avoided.
- *Safer Assessment* integrates safety into daily classroom routines of teaching, learning, assessment, and homework.
  - *Feedback Fades Fear* recognizes the stress created when everything students do counts for grades. Consider a balance of helpful, formative feedback versus hardcore evaluations in your class to take pressure off, where possible.
  - *Revealing the Target* provides clear, student-friendly, assessment criteria *before* students begin a learning cycle to lessen anxiety and increase chances for success.
- *Life Support* is making a personal, private check-in with a student for two minutes a day, for five to ten days in a row, helping them deal with a difficulty.[9] This could be someone who seems to be struggling, or any student that really needs a connection. These check-ins can begin by letting the student talk about a neutral topic, rather than jumping into asking how they are doing personally.
- *Safety Nets* are student help lines, district services, and community agencies that provide a world of support from free counseling to financial aid. These organizations often provide single-page fact sheets that can be posted on a classroom wall under a brightly lettered "Safety Nets" title. Connect with your school social worker, counselor, or psychologist for recommendations of school and community resources to be included. Safety nets supplement, but do not replace, the need for teachers to refer and report students in need (see p. 38).
- *Welcome Graffiti* are positive, inclusive quotes, or translations of welcoming phrases, which help all students feel welcomed and represented at school. These can be drawn by students outside using sidewalk chalk, posted in the halls, or captured and tagged to school social media.

3

SOCIAL WELL-BEING

Relationships, Community, and Belonging

"The foundation of what makes lives go well is not the individual, but the quality of our relationships; the development of trust, the giving and receiving of love, and the myriad ways in which relationships can be life-enhancing."

—Felicia Huppert

One of the most transformative practices of well-being is a simple thought experiment. To try it now, follow the steps below in a heartfelt way.[1]

1. Bring to mind one of the happiest, most satisfying moments of your life.
2. Engage your senses to see, hear, and feel the experience with vividness and emotion.
3. With memory glowing inside you, *hold it close* for a minute. Feel it warm and marinate your entire being. Let it sink deeply into your heart.

How was that? Chances are there is a warmer feeling than a minute ago. It's also likely your happy moment involved others or was shared with others in some way. In fact, connection is so crucial that humans have sophisticated social skills that set us apart from other species.[2]

Brené Brown has explored the underpinnings of belonging and found that it hinges on self-acceptance, one of many social skills that can be practiced in class.[3] This practice is key, as most students spend significant social time online, which fails to develop interpersonal skills and can even subvert self-acceptance. Classrooms, being full of humans, are ideal places to cultivate critical social skills.

The benefits of belonging are rich and durable, going beyond simple love, support, and sharing—reaching deeply into multiple domains of wellness:

- healthier lifestyle behaviors, faster healing, and longer physical life;[4]
- reduced mental stress and fewer depressive symptoms;[5]
- greater life satisfaction and emotional fulfillment;[6] and
- stronger meaning and identity in being part of something larger.[7]

WELL-BEING IS SOCIAL

Healthy connections are not just a *source* of well-being, they are also a vehicle for *sharing* it. A twenty-year, large-scale study of happiness in social networks found that relationships contributed to the flow of wellness in those networks.[8] In other words, we benefit from connection *and* from the wellness of those with whom we connect. This positive "network effect" happens across all social ties or connections, extends to three degrees of separation, and endures years into the future. Classroom relationships benefit both learning and wellness.[9] Researcher Trudi Norman-Murch explains: "All learning takes place in the context of relationships and is critically affected by the quality of those relationships."[10]

Here's another thought experiment that reveals the synergy of social wellness. Consider that one teacher (or student) alone has a single relationship—with themselves. Putting teacher and student together makes three relationships. Adding a second student makes six, and so on. A class of thirty plus a teacher has 496 possible connections. Add thousands more beyond the classroom and the vast well of social potential becomes clear.

For a final thought experiment, consider some of the most important relationships you have had in schools, whether with staff or students or others. How have these relationships changed you, and impacted on your wellness? Can you even count them all?

This myriad of relationships formed in the school years can be life-defining—or life-crushing. While social-emotional learning (SEL) standards are used in about half of U.S. districts (mostly in primary), many schools have no explicit learning around human connection.[11] Teachers also need training to facilitate such learning, and for their personal social thriving. Teacher wellness, critical in its own right, is a catalyst for a healthy, happy classroom.

Well-being is a shared mission, with individual and collective wellness (for students and staff) as one seamless endeavor. The fact that wellness is also shared across social connections only makes this more true. Teachers who can nurture healthy social ties and belonging expand everyone's capacity to connect in the classroom and beyond. The ultimate experiment is to dig into social well-being activities and help community, relationships, and belonging flourish.

Key Messages

- Social well-being is perhaps the most fundamental domain of human wellness.
- Benefits of connection and belonging stretch across every domain of well-being.
- Enduring wellness is developed and shared within social networks.

SOCIAL WELL-BEING ACTIVITIES

Circle Check-Ins (Main Move)

> "In the Circle we are all equal. When in the Circle, no one is in front of you and no one is behind you. No one is above you. No one is below you. The Sacred Circle is designed to create unity."
>
> —Dave Yakima Chief Wakinyan

The circle is at once a powerful and familiar classroom tradition stretching from kindergarten to the highest levels of learning, rooted in Indigenous traditions. Whether for community-building, learning, or restoring peace, circles build classroom relationships and deepen trust. The social capital generated from circles is not only vital for well-being, but contributes to social–emotional growth, reduced suspensions, and improved school climate.[12]

Beyond these benefits, circles are also catalysts for personal and social shifts. Educators who use circles long enough realize this potential:

- *In the first classroom circle of the year, Ben had his arms crossed, earbuds in, hood up, face scowling, and seat pushed back from the rest of the circle. After a half-dozen circles, he was transformed: uncrossing, unplugging, opening up, and checking in with a smile.*
- *Juliana didn't expect the staff meeting to be in a circle, or to hear colleagues opening up in ways they never had before. But when the guest facilitator, Adam, shared that his clinic helped those impacted by childhood sexual abuse, Juliana's heart skipped a beat. After the circle closed, after most had left, and after years of silence, Juliana found herself face-to-face with Adam, who met her silent gaze, and knew.*
- *Jenn's grade-8 science class was more than a handful. One of her early circles ended abruptly with the talking piece hurled across the circle. After developing agreements, and building capacity in small circles for months, the entire class responded authentically and peacefully in a whole class circle check-in: a first, but not a last.*
- *The grade-7 team at Central PS were very close, having eaten lunch together for seventeen years, but when they shared in a circle what they valued and cherished about each other, as they had never done before, they brought themselves to tears.*

A circle's power begins with its geometry. Classroom rows with a teacher desk upfront can disconnect and disempower, but circles let everyone make eye contact and sit equidistant from the center, sharing power. Indeed, since no one is placed in front of, or behind another, feelings,

SOCIAL WELL-BEING

learning, and decisions can arise from any point on the circumference. The entire group is responsible for keeping the circle in a good way, and for the overall group harmony.

Harmonious circles develop key wellness qualities such as *authenticity, caring, connection, empathy, equanimity, flexibility, listening, openness, optimism, presence, sensitivity, vulnerability, and wholeness.* These aspects may be felt immediately by simply sitting in a circle and gazing with each person silently, as well as in circle activities. Verbally acknowledge these qualities when they arise to encourage even more of them.

Any quality deeply actualized in one person can be shared directly with everyone in the circle. The mechanisms for this transmission include social contagion and emotional mimicry, which boost connection and social rapport as well as providing an index for empathy.[13] For example, genuine authenticity has a flavor and feel that is clearly apparent to all present. This flavor sparks authenticity in others, imbuing the circle in a palpable ring of truth. Exploring and debriefing these qualities as they arise in circles helps with their germination and development.

Circle participation over time develops these qualities, along with classroom relationships, collectively referred to as a circle's *capacity*. This activity introduces a safe and foundational circle practice requiring little or no capacity: the community circle check-in. As circle capacity increases, activities requiring higher trust, and with a correspondingly higher potential for well-being, are possible. Infinite variations of circling include energizers (p. 229), games (p. 197), learning circles (p. 171), fishbowls (p. 190), and restorative circles (p. 136).

If you have never facilitated a circle, just begin. But begin with the wholehearted intention to cultivate circle qualities, and let these qualities emanate from everything you do. As your circles with students evolve in harmony and wellness, see what magic can arise.

Summary: Use check-in questions in a circle to build community, trust, and relationships.
Time: 5–20 minutes
Trust Required: Varies

1. *Prep* (1 minute): On hearing "circle up please," students move furniture quietly and put away devices and bags. Circles can happen in the classroom, hall, outdoors, or anywhere there is space. Students may sit on the desks, on the floor, or stand up—it's still a circle. Some optional preparations may feel helpful or inviting:
   a. *Prepare a timer* with a soft chime to keep talk time balanced and allow students to practice the timekeeper role using a phone or app.
   b. *Provide fidget toys or manipulatives* such as pipe cleaners, squish balls or plastic toys to give students something to occupy their hands and inspire prompts (e.g., "I feel like this [toy or pipe cleaner shape] right now because . . .").
   c. *Co-create a talking piece* with the class, perhaps using a plushie initialed by each student, or a branch with the favorite sayings of each student attached.
   d. *Add a centerpiece* such as a stone, flameless candle, inspirational quotation of the day, or thumball to give a central focus, and aid in placing chairs.
   e. *Tune the circle* by adding or removing chairs as needed, closing gaps, and adjusting the shape so everyone can make eye contact. You may leave one chair empty to represent those not present.
2. *Open* (2 minutes): Explain anything new, if needed (e.g., different purpose for the circle or a new student in class). Transparency about your intentions as to *why* the circle is happening is important, as the class may assume a circle is only held after something has gone wrong. Consider whether a moment of mindfulness (p. 145) can ground the group.

3. *Check-In Prompt* (1 minute): Select a prompt (see table 3.1) that reflects the trust level of the group. Speak the prompt to the circle, and model how to respond by going first, sharing authentically in the time frame desired. This helps participants feel safer, get a sense of how much time to take, and normalizes the practice of vulnerability.
4. *Student Responses* (3–10 minutes): While circles are organic and can travel in many directions, two basic formats are sequential rounds and non-sequential sharing.
    a. *Sequential rounds* pass the right to speak (and talking piece if used) to the adjacent person, counterclockwise or clockwise depending on tradition, until everyone has had the opportunity to say something. Rounds can take time, so time limits can be helpful, while sometimes no limit will feel right.
    b. *Non-sequential sharing* lets participants indicate with a hand signal that they wish to speak. If used, the talking piece is passed to that person, so they can speak or respond, then wait silently for the next student to indicate a desire to share.

    Discussions sometimes move in unplanned yet wonderful directions. Don't hesitate to follow topical tangents that seem fruitful or deepen the sharing with multiple rounds.
5. *Close/Debrief* (0–2 minutes): The facilitator expresses gratitude, with an optional round to let participants say one word they are feeling, closing the circle in a good way. Standard debrief questions (see p. 16) may also be used at this time, likely with a non-sequential format. This is also an opportunity to acknowledge any circle *qualities* that were felt.
6. *Safety*: Basic cooperation is required to begin a circle. The main trust consideration depends on the check-in question used. In the early days of building trust and community, the following may help create a safer circle environment:
    a. Ease in with students first sitting behind desks, perhaps in a wider semicircle, then gradually close the circle and

remove desks. Smaller circles of three or four may also help prepare students for a large circle experience. Post a sign on the door "Circle in progress" to reflect circle sacredness and privacy.

b. Co-create circle agreements (see p. 44), and consider including some mainstays: right to pass/participate (*participation*); eyes/ears/hearts open (*listening*); devices away (*presence*); speak what is true, necessary, and kind (see p. 84); share your own experience, not that of others (*confidentiality*).

c. Share first as a teacher to ease the way for others and use a talking piece.

d. Share facilitation with students allowing them to create circle questions, and ultimately transition to having no facilitator.

Table 3.1. Check-In Prompts

Low Trust Required	*Medium Trust Required*	*High Trust Required*
• A brag and a drag . . .	• A moment I'd relive . . .	• A big event in my life . . .
• Desert island [song, book, film, etc.] . . .	• A memory from time in nature . . .	• A challenge for me is . . .
• A job I would like . . .	• A dream I have . . .	• A change I'd like to see . . .
• A place I'd go . . .	• A present I got/gave . . .	• A dream I have had . . .
• A superpower I'd like . . .	• Recently, this happened . . .	• A childhood memory . . .
• An exciting experience . . .	• In my free time, I . . .	• A mistake I made . . .
• I'm a [dog/cat, indoor/outdoor] person . . .	• A rose, bud, and thorn for me right now . . .	• Something I learned the hard way . . .
• My favorite [band, color, class, film, food, hobby, music, number, pet, season, smell] is . . . because . . .	• When I was younger . . .	• A passion of mine . . .
	• A person that makes me feel good is . . .	• A person that impacted me . . .
	• A time when I was [happy, upset, wise, peaceful, uncertain] . . .	• A school memory . . .
• I am grateful for . . .	• I get in a flow doing . . .	• A special possession . . .
• I'm lucky that . . .	• If I need advice . . .	• A time when I was [afraid, mad, brilliant, sad, embarrassed, proud, generous, selfish, loving, foolish] . . .
• I celebrate . . .	• If I could ask a question of anyone who ever lived . . .	• I matter because . . .
• I laugh when . . .	• I destress by . . .	• For me, the word home . . .
• A creative outlet . . .	• I was influenced by . . .	• It hurts when . . .
• I recharge by . . .	• My happy place . . .	• I hurt someone when . . .
• If I had a day off . . .	• I'm different . . .	• My relationship with my family . . .
• If I was an animal . . .		
• Life's easier when . . .		
• Someone I admire . . .		

SOCIAL WELL-BEING

Low Trust Required	Medium Trust Required	High Trust Required
• Something I want to create . . .	• My superpower . . .	• What I deeply love . . .
• You're awesome if . . .	• My online life . . .	• Love feels like . . .
• I wouldn't change . . .	• My healthy habit . . .	• What I love about me . . .
• Something new . . .	• I tried something new . . .	• A turning point for me . . .
• Something true . . .	• A good friend . . .	• A best friend might say I'm . . .
• Three words for right now . . .	• Love or be loved?	• I am stressed out by . . .
• One thing I'm sure about . . .	• When I get older . . .	• I broke a rule . . .
• I worked hard . . .	• A talent I have . . .	• Giving up is good when . . .
• I look forward to . . .	• I grew up . . .	• I'm outside my comfort zone . . .
• I prioritize . . .	• About my name . . .	• The hardest thing about school . . .
• I want . . .	• My family . . .	• My big moment this year . . .
• An ideal day . . .	• Something I do well. . .	• My guilty pleasure . . .
• I wonder . . .	• I respect . . . because . . .	• My greatest fear . . .
• My treasure . . .	• I'd tell the world . . .	• A peak, a valley, and a twist in my journey . . .
	• Three words about me . . .	• A person who impacted me . . .
	• My motto . . .	• Someone or something I miss . . .
		• Something I created . . .
		• Something I lost or found was . . .
		• Something I'm holding onto . . .
		• Most people don't know about me . . .
		• What's meaningful for me . . .
		• When someone is (angry, caring, distracted, upset, loving etc.) I . . .
		• The three most important words . . .

Keywords: caring, choice, circle, collaborative, empower, foundational, get-to-know, icebreaker, identity, short-'n'-safe, social, space

Caring Adult Connections for Every Student

> "The goal isn't just to support kids academically, it's about building positive relationships and helping students grow as human beings."
>
> —Paul Dawson

Students can fall through the cracks at any school, but at a large high school of 2000, Vice Principal Paul Dawson knew the risk was even greater. Paul led the staff through a process to create a connection between each youth and at least one caring adult in the building. He knew that positive adult-student relationships not only support academic success for students, but contribute to belonging, emotional health, and well-being.[14]

> **Summary**: Staff review student photos to identify and connect with potentially isolated students.
> **Time**: 60+ minutes
> **Trust Required**: Low
>
> 1. *Prep*: Gather student photos and share with staff digitally or print many per page. The photos can be laid out at a staff meeting or shared online for staff to access and edit.
> 2. *Launch* (5 minutes): This strategy is best initiated a month or so after the first day of school, to allow some adult-student connections to form. Lead off with some research or learning on the importance of student-staff relationships and school belonging perhaps using the citations provided.
> 3. *Check Students* (10–20 minutes): Staff scan the photos and write their name (or place a check mark) beside any student with which they have a significant connection. A connection is more than just having the student in a class and could be
>   a. readily recognizing the student by name and face;
>   b. having spoken to the student more than once; and/or
>   c. having some other connection personally, or from a club or team.

4. *Collate Unconnected Students* (10 minutes): Students *without* a caring adult connection are identified. This may be 10 percent of the student body, though this varies greatly.
5. *Intentional Connections* (5 minutes): Staff members may then volunteer to become a caring adult connection for (an) identified student(s). Teachers who have the student in a class are an obvious start, but any adult staff can commit to getting to know this student. Assigning one student per staff member may suffice, although some teachers may offer to take on more depending on their class lists. The matching process can be supported with the school team of administration, guidance or special education as needed.
6. *Build Connections* (varies): Teachers make a natural effort to establish student connections. Here are three simple, research-supported approaches to do this:
   a. Greeting students in halls and at doorways (see "Doorways to Connection," p. 68).
   b. Discovering similarities between teacher and student (Gehlbach et al., 2016).
   c. Getting to know what is unique about each student (Vidourek and King, 2014).
7. *Follow-Up* (30 minutes): In the weeks following the photo review, follow-up meetings (or online updates) can be arranged to manage evolving connections. Encourage teachers to put forward names of students with whom they have not yet connected so backup can be arranged. Staff can also share stories about *how* they connected to give ideas. Attendance or achievement for these students can be compared pre- and post-process. Vice Principal Dawson found significant gains in both areas for supported students. A small reward or gratitude can be provided to teachers as a thank you for the extra effort they are making.
8. *Safety*: Staff do not share the strategy itself with students but interact naturally with those for whom they have volunteered to become a caring adult.

9. *Schoolwide Extension*: This activity is a natural schoolwide initiative and optimally effective as such. The scope can also be limited to a single grade or other student cohort if student needs dictate, or time and resources are limited.

Keywords: caring, collaborative, get-to-know, lifeplay, safety, schoolwide, social, support

Catching Goodness: Elevation

Seeing the essential goodness of others can be a profound and moving experience, as described by Thomas Merton, American monk and author: "I suddenly saw the secret beauty of their hearts. . . . If only we could see each other that way all the time."[15] Noticing goodness does more than acknowledge, it also inspires the doer, who (in the words of Nelson Mandela) "often act the better because of it." It also turns out that *observers* of prosocial behavior (or any act of moral beauty) experience a constellation of positive feelings, even when they aren't the beneficiary of the good deed. This dynamic of *elevation* elicits hope, optimism, and moral inspiration, inspiring those who witness good deeds with the desire to connect, help others, and be better people.[16]

The sharing of witnessed events has a similar effect, whether those involved are socially connected or not.[17] All these forms of elevation create a blanket of benevolence, warming the entire community with joy, selflessness, and the desire to do good things.

In this activity, classroom social capital is fostered through catching goodness in two ways. The first "catching" is to record or write down good deeds on a public display. The second, longer lasting "catching" is to capture feelings of elevation in the heart, merging them with the inherent goodness already there (see self-directed neuroplasticity, p. 156, for more on this).

Creating a structured way to notice excellence in others (whether a caring peer, inspiring teacher, or anyone doing a selfless act) positively impacts student behavior, relationships, and well-being.[18] The mixture of gratitude and admiration that comes with elevation doesn't just make classrooms happier, it inspires everyone in them to be better and do better.

Summary: Notice, post and acknowledge positive or prosocial acts.
Time: 20 minutes
Trust Required: Low

1. *Prep* (10 minutes): Gather blank sticky notes or copy preprinted slips (figure 3.1), and prepare a wall, bulletin board or poster to display the notes. The activity can also be done electronically in any collaborative online space.
2. *Catch* (over several weeks): Students and teachers are encouraged to write down good deeds or virtuous acts of moral beauty that they witness in the classroom or school (e.g., caring, honesty, helping) using a blank sticky note or preprinted slip (see figure 3.1). Building a virtues vocabulary may be a helpful aid to this activity (see p. 31).

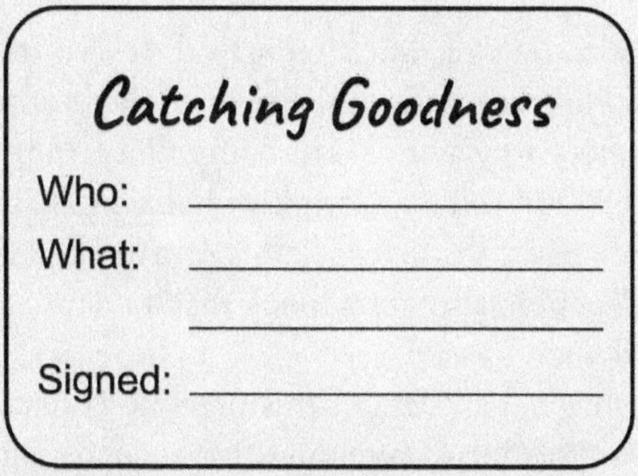

Catching Goodness
Who: _____
What: _____
_____
Signed: _____

Figure 3.1. Catching Goodness

3. *Share* (1 minute): Post these slips to a "Catching Goodness" wall, bulletin board or poster displayed prominently in class (see schoolwide extension below for other options).
4. *Debrief* (5 minutes): Visit the board periodically to review new posts, asking observers to describe what they saw and any related feelings felt (see *debriefing*, p. 13, for more).
5. *Safety*: As with any public display, monitor posts regularly.

6. *Lifeplay*: Distribute copies of the preprinted slips as cards and invite students to note acts of moral beauty outside school. Debrief the impact of doing this often.
7. *Schoolwide Extension*: Create a central "Catching Goodness" display in a prominent place within the school or on the school website. Share positive acts at announcements or any larger gathering. Ensure all staff *and students* can contribute, since the mechanism of elevation will swell with more eyes and ears capturing good deeds. Staff can also name and claim strengths they see in others within their staff group.

Keywords: caring, cognitive, emotional, eudaimonia, gratitude, hedonia, schoolwide, social, space

Doorways to Connection

It feels great to be welcomed on arrival. It also feels great to be the welcomer. Greeting students at the door of the classroom (or school) is a simple but effective way to boost community, improve academic engagement time,[19] and reduce disruptive behavior.[20] By transforming the jostling between classes into a socially positive class start, learning time is improved. Teachers also get a quick read on student moods that may otherwise have been missed.

One of the magical aspects of this practice is that it actually *creates* time. For a class of thirty, spending five seconds with each student is more than made up for with better quality learning time and reduced time spent dealing with behavior during class.

But the best byproduct of this activity is goodwill. Lisa Fipps writes about the magical powers of a librarian greeting students in her body-positive verse novel *Starfish*: "She's the first person to smile at me today. The first to make me feel wanted. Understood."[21]

As students gladden on hearing a welcome, the welcomer also warms, for in greeting others, we are greeted in return. Imagine that each interaction is a precious moment that will never come again, for that's exactly what it is.

Summary: Stand at the door to greet students warmly and personally as they enter class.
Time: 3 minutes
Trust Required: Low

1. *Greet*: Stand beside the doorway to class and greet students in a variety of ways, recognizing the uniqueness of each interaction.
   a. *Facial expressions:* eye contact, smile, nod, wink.
   b. *Non-verbal signals*: thumbs-up, high-five, fist/elbow bump, handshake, bow, wave of arm, hand on heart, clap, jazz hands, happy dance.
   c. *Verbal greetings*: "hello," "hey," "hi," or a greeting in the student's language.
   d. *Acknowledgements*: "good to see you," "thank you for coming to class," "glad you are here" or speaking the student's name brightly—"Kishanth!!!"
   e. *Encouragement*: "nice shirt/shoes/hat," "thanks for bringing your stuff today."
   f. *Prompts*: "what's for lunch today?" or "did you get a haircut?" If you ask "how's it going?," take the time to hear their reply (see p. 196 for more).
2. *Safety*: Learn how different students would like to be greeted by asking them. Where there is a significant height differential between teacher and students, use a chair to meet the students at their level. When asking questions such as "what's for lunch today?," be attuned to the responses and the lived experiences that are coming through the door.
3. *Schoolwide Extension*: This initiative is easily scaled to include the whole staff, or an entire grade. When a majority of staff values relationship-building, there is a correspondingly pro-social and pro-learning impact. Consider flexing the time span, doing a one-week blitz, focusing on a particular cohort, or switching grades on different days. Another variation involves staff greeting any student (including those not in their

classes) by standing in hallways. School leaders who do this routinely and genuinely validate positive inclusion for all in a huge way.

Keywords: caring, emotional, get-to-know, identity, prep-free, schoolwide, social, short-'n'-safe, time-maker

Mindful Listening

"There is no concept of justice in Cree culture. The nearest word is kintohpatatin, which loosely translates to 'you've been listened to.' But kintohpatatin is richer than justice—really it means you've been listened to by someone compassionate and fair, and your needs will be taken seriously."[22]

—Edmund Metatawabin

Edmund Metatawabin, author, advocate for residential school survivors, and member of the Order of Canada, describes the power of serious listening. While mindfulness is not typically seen as a social endeavor, mindful listening—with absolute presence and compassion—takes connection to a new level. When we listen with our ears, eyes, bodies, and hearts, the speaker feels supported to share deeply. As a listener's capacities develop, they become more willing to be changed by the words heard without needing to jump in. Contrast this with the typical experience of "listening" where there is distraction, thinking of what to say next or interrupting.

The traditional Chinese character for listen (ting 聽, see figure 3.2) encompasses many of these aspects: wrapping your ear around the speaker (as though they were a king), listening with ten eyes (full attention) and one heart (wholeheartedly). Listening with the whole being allows us to also hear what is arising *within ourselves*. Mindful listening isn't just listening to the other in a non-reactive and accepting way but also involves listening to our own experience. The result can be deeper

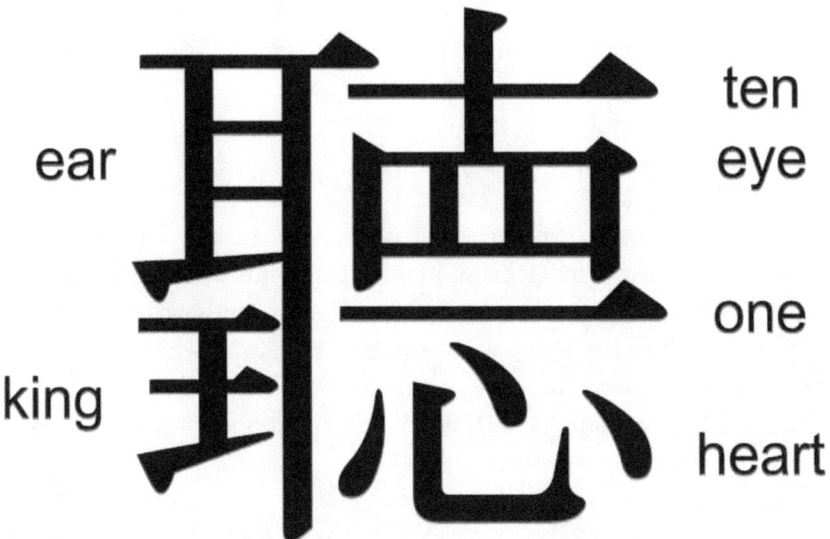

Figure 3.2. Listen in Traditional Chinese

sharing, stronger connections, and a healthy intimacy in any interaction. Listening mindfully can be practiced with students, colleagues, family, or friends. The key to developing this rare and beautiful skill is to make it a lifelong practice, not a one-time activity.

After an all-day workshop, a participant asked the facilitator about applying the learning to their role. Their question turned into a venting of frustrations about this role, but the facilitator didn't interrupt. Instead, they stopped packing their things and deeply listened. As the participant went on, the entire group cleared away and left, but the facilitator stayed present, saying nothing. Ultimately, the venting trailed off, and the participant, feeling utterly heard, brushed away a tear, gave the facilitator a quick embrace, and left with a smile.

As deep listening is a core aspect of deep connection, it has the potential to transform relationships and daily interactions from the mundane to the sacred. Be open to the possibilities of listening lovingly with the whole being, and see what can be revealed, or healed.

Summary: Listen with body, mind, heart, and soul—practice often.
Time: 20 minutes
Trust Required: Medium

1. *Prep*: Provide prompts the day before so students can prepare a response, especially multilingual students learning English.
2. *Warmup* (1 minute): Give everyone 30 seconds to listen to the sounds in the room as a warmup. Brainstorm what "deep listening" means to students, which *may* include the following:
    a. Giving complete attention, putting phones and other gear away.
    b. Turning to face the person in an open way (listening with the body).
    c. Making eye contact and taking in body language (listening with the eyes).
    d. Remaining silent and attentive to their words (listening with the ears).
    e. Feeling what is shared in your body (listening with the heart).
    f. Not interrupting or responding in any way, even if you really want to.
    g. Listening to whatever might be arising inside *you* as you listen.
3. *Explain and Prompt* (4 minutes): Pair up students and give them a prompt (see table 3.1) such as "a brag and a drag for me right now is . . ." Explain that each partner will be speaking *uninterrupted for two full minutes* in response to this prompt, while the other person listens mindfully. Give some time for students to absorb this and consider what they might talk about. Let them know that it is okay to pause or trail off; their partner will listen silently for the full two minutes and won't interrupt, just nodding or giving non-verbal cues. Reinforce the brainstormed aspects of deep listening before beginning.

SOCIAL WELL-BEING

4. *Speaking and Listening* (5 minutes): Use a timer and cue each stage below.
   a. Person A Shares (2 minutes): person A speaks to the prompt, B mindfully listens.
   b. Silent Pause (30 seconds): invite everyone to pause and reflect silently.
   c. Person B Shares (2 minutes): person B speaks to the prompt, A mindfully listens.
   d. Silent Pause (30 seconds): invite the group to pause and reflect silently.
5. *Partner Debrief* (3 minutes): Partners now share freely with each other about their experiences, both from a listening and speaking point of view.
6. *Whole Group Debrief* (7 minutes): Consider the following prompts to help debrief.
   a. Use any of the standard debrief questions (see p. 16).
   b. How did it feel to be a mindful listener?
   c. How did it feel to be sharing while someone listened deeply without speaking?
   d. Did you judge yourself (or the other) at any time for not responding back?
7. *"Is There More?"* (Optional): When a speaker pauses, the listener can remain in loving presence, giving them silent permission to go on. After a longer pause, the listener may simply ask, "Is there more?" Repeated cycles of listening and asking "Is there more?" may reveal previously undiscovered depths in the interaction. This query can be used for any class discussion or activity that explores deeper issues.
8. *Lifeplay*: One experience may be informative, but a lifetime of practicing is transformative. Invite the class to use mindful listening with others in their personal lives, and report back on the experience. Commit to doing this yourself as the teacher as well. Repeat the practice in class periodically to remind students to use the practice and debrief any lifeplay to see how things are going. As mindful listening capacity

grows, it will naturally start to permeate life at school, home, and beyond. One lifeplay challenge could be to mindfully listen to a family member or loved one using the "Is there more?" option. Another lifeplay invitation is to notice how the choice to listen mindfully is an *action* that changes the nature of the *interaction*. Debriefing is vital to refresh the practice but also to reveal the magic and meaning inherent in mindful listening.

9. *Safety*: A depth of listening evokes a corresponding depth of sharing, which brings up challenging thoughts and emotions for some. Remind students of confidentiality, and stay attuned and supportive to those who may be deeply affected by the experience.
10. *Integration Strategy*: Use a curriculum-related prompt in step 3 above as part of regular classroom discussions or partner work to bring new depths of learning and social connection. In this way, the vital skill of listening can be practiced while teaching mathematics, social studies, the arts, or any subject. Mindful listening and silent reflection breathes vital spaces into packed learning. As music is the space between the notes, so too does meaning and learning inhabit the sacred pauses in classrooms.

Keywords: card, caring, get-to-know, integration, lifeplay, mindfulness, prep-free, restorative, social, short-n'-safe, spiritual

Mingle Bingo

A combination of movement, bingo, and learning silly things about each other makes this activity a great ice breaker for students and staff. Mingle bingo can be adapted as a learning activity as well (see integration strategy below). We are inherently social creatures, so connection-oriented activities increase engagement while building social capital.

Summary: Classmates move freely, looking for others to fill their bingo card.
Time: 15 minutes
Trust Required: Low

1. *Prep* (5 minutes): Prepare and copy cards for each participant, or distribute blank cards and let participants write their own questions. Small prizes add to the fun.
2. *Mingle* (10 minutes): No bingo caller is required, students simply mingle in the group, looking for someone who can answer "yes" to any question on their bingo card.
   a. Match: When a person matches something on a card, that person initials the square.
   b. BINGO: The first student to have five squares signed in a line wins. This can be extended to recognize multiple bingos, two lines, or a full card, keeping the game going depending on time available. For groups of twenty-five or more, getting a full card might become the aim.
3. *Integration Strategy*: Replace the squares with curriculum-related prompts, questions, or mini-problems. Students then answer questions, complete mini-tasks, or have short discussions with a variety of partners related to the current unit.
4. *Schoolwide Extension*: Play mingle bingo with staff as a get-to-know activity.
5. *Safety*: While cards are typically pre-filled for convenience, having them blank allows participants to choose their own questions, adding a layer of student choice and voice.

Keywords: choice, collaborative, get-to-know, hedonia, icebreaker, identity, integration, physical, schoolwide, social, short-'n'-safe

Table 3.2. Mingle Bingo Example Card

Mingle Bingo				
Born in another country.	Has worn more than one cast in their life.	Left handed.	Likes dancing.	Played a sport in school.
Read a book in the past month.	Has exactly two siblings.	Favorite food is a vegetable.	Last name has an "R" in it.	Has two or more pets.
Plays video games.	Born in September.	FREE	Has been in a play.	Wearing something green.
Can play a musical instrument.	Likes roller coasters.	Has no siblings.	Favorite subject is art.	Afraid of spiders.
Has volunteered for a charity.	Danced at a wedding.	Meditates.	Eats sushi.	Keeps a journal.

Partner Drawing

> "Creating together helps people organize and externalize thoughts and feelings that may be otherwise difficult to articulate. The guided creative process, as well as the end product, can be used to enhance a person's emotional, spiritual, social, cognitive, and physical well-being."
>
> —Ashtyn Ford

The creative arts have a vast potential for developing the emotional, cognitive, and meaning-making domains of well-being. This activity could benefit any of these areas, but its social aspect stands out. When two people create together in silence, their ideas and feelings are shared in ways that transcend words. Silence and presence are key aspects to bringing a transformative potential to this activity. Partner drawing may be part of an arts program as an integration strategy or experienced as a stand-alone wellness activity in any class.

Summary: Two people create art together by taking turns drawing then debriefing.
Time: 10 minutes
Trust Required: Low

1. *Prep*: Gather recycled paper (good on one side) and art materials or personal whiteboards (1 per pair) and dry-erase markers. Digital tools can also work although an unplugged experience is desirable.
2. *Setup* (1 minute): Pair students (see p. 31) with a blank sheet/board for each pair.
3. *Explanation* (2 minutes): Explain that students will take turns making a sketch, mark, or part of a drawing on the page. Have them start with something small, and then take turns adding to what is already there—gradually. Drawing skill is *not* the focus of the activity. The emphasis is to authentically express whatever wants to show up on the page, while connecting with another person through art. Students will remain silent during the entire drawing phase. Students mutually agree with a silent nod when the art is finished.
4. *Pause* (30 seconds): Lead a stretch of silent grounding, inviting students to look at the blank sheet together.
5. *Drawing Phase* (3 minutes): One student draws briefly and pauses. The other student may then add to the drawing in turn and pause themselves. This is repeated for a few minutes, or until the pair agrees their art is complete.
6. *Silent Reflection* (30 seconds): Both reflect silently on the shared creation.
7. *Debrief* (3 minutes)
   a. Pairs: debrief using the standard questions (see p. 16)
   b. Whole class: ask if anyone would like to tell the story of their picture.
8. *Safety*: As with any activity where internal feelings may surface, watch for students who may have a challenging experience. See p. 21 for more on trauma-informed activity.

Keywords: choice, cognitive, collaborative, creative, emotional, icebreaker, integration, social, short-'n'-safe

Seeing and Sharing the Goodness

> "To see the goodness is to do what Einstein called 'widening our circle of compassion': the well-wishing or loving-kindness that sees the original innocence, the dignity, the beauty of another, and also is in touch with that same secret beauty, that original innocence, in oneself."[23]
>
> —Jack Kornfield

Jack Kornfield is a beloved teacher of mindfulness and loving kindness who shares stories of well-being. One involved a math teacher who asked her students to see the goodness in each other. She gave them blank class lists on which they wrote down what they admired or liked about each other student in the class. She collected these, cut them up, and reassembled them so each student could read the kind, loving words written for them by their classmates.

Years later, the teacher got a phone call from the mother of one student, Paul, who told her that Paul had died in military action. The mother also said the teacher had been Paul's favorite, and she invited her to the memorial service. At the service, with other classmates gathered, Paul's mother held up a tattered piece of paper, one of a few things found on his body. The paper had been folded and unfolded many times, and she unfolded it one more time to read aloud the loving words shared by Paul's classmates. The teacher watched as the others from the class reached into their pockets and purses to draw out their own lists of goodness, which they had carried with them from that classroom so many years ago.

Summary: Students share and receive written words of kindness with classmates.
Time: 30 minutes
Trust Required: Medium

1. *Prep*: Print and distribute a blank class list to each student, or use a digital survey tool and ensure students have devices. The online option greatly facilitates the summarizing process and preserves anonymity by avoiding handwriting but is less personal.

2. *Writing Kindness* (10 minutes): Explain the process using something like the following script. "We often see good things in others, but we may not realize the good things others see in us. Today we're going to share some good things about each other. Write down something *kind, good, positive,* or *admirable* about every other student in the class. I will review these and then you will get a summary of what others have said about you. It's important that we keep the process anonymous so everyone feels safe to share."
3. *Collate* (10+ minutes): Collect and review the comments. Assemble comments for each student on one page with their name at the top or compile using an online form.
4. *Share Back* (5 minutes): When sharing these precious comments with students, reiterate the importance of respecting the anonymity of the process, and the preciousness of kind words shared honestly. A circle process could respect the import of the process.
5. *Debrief* (5 minutes): Begin with the default debrief questions, and see where the dialogue goes, or use these prompts:
    a. How does it feel to read the comments written about you?
    b. How was it for you to share something good about another person?
    c. Do you think you could write the same list about yourself? Why or why not?
6. *Safety*: Ensure students have reached some depth of knowing each other so that comments can be meaningful and authentic. Emphasize the anonymity requirement, so students can feel more free and honest with what they say and to avoid comparisons. Review the comments before distribution to ensure each student has comments and that all the comments are kind and caring.

Keywords: caring, collaborative, emotional, gratitude, hedonia, social

Thumball Sharing

> "I could put my thumb up to a window and completely hide the Earth. I thought, 'Everything I've ever known is behind my thumb.'"
>
> —Jim Lovell

A great deal can be revealed—or hidden—behind a thumb held over a globe. And to play catch with a ball brings a refreshing lightness to the formality of school. These are the basic elements of using a *thumball*: having some fun in the classroom while shining a light on who is in that room. Through a variety of get-to-know-you questions printed on a ball, students can share about themselves and learn about others in turn.

Most thumballs have questions written on them that require only a low level of trust, to increase safety and fun. Table 3.3 provides some sensible starting points. These prompts are brief enough to fit on a ball. Although some students may appreciate, or even enjoy, the vulnerability of deeper questions, others may feel challenged with sensitive topics.

The essence of playing ball is lightness and fun. Consider using deeper prompts as your classroom trust develops and keep in mind that *any* topic or question might potentially bring up challenging thoughts for a particular student. Let the arc and delight of each toss, catch, or miss, sprinkled with discovering who is in the room, cultivate fun, relaxation, and closeness that is so vital for social well-being.

Summary: Students take turns catching a ball then responding to a prompt written on it.
Time: 5–10 minutes
Trust Required: Low (or varies)

1. *Prep*: Find any soft, easily catchable ball and write question prompts using the suggestions in table 3.3. Although preprinted thumballs may be purchased, teachers can make use of a compromised soccer ball or volleyball, since deflated balls are easier to catch. Alternatively, any plush ball that can take a permanent marker works well. Given enough blank balls, students could create their own thumballs, providing student ownership and voice. For complete flexibility, create

a thumball with numbers only and project sets of questions as numbered lists, allowing for a variety of uses. Consider creating one special thumball dedicated to relationship-building.
2. *Model Catching and Responding* (1 minute): Begin by emphasizing the ball as a talking piece, with attention and speaking rights granted to the ball holder.
   a. Hold out two open hands to indicate a willingness to receive the ball.
   b. Demonstrate tossing the ball gently to oneself, catching with two hands. Show how the thumb and/or fingers point to possible questions, offering choice.
   c. Model responding by reading out a question and giving an authentic, on-the-fly response using the time frame desired.
3. Circulate the thumball (5–10 minutes): Invite students to hold out two open hands, and begin passing the thumball, which will naturally prompt a response and be passed along. Anyone not holding the ball listens to responses without cross-talk and holds their hands out to receive the ball. Some possible variations and additions follow:
   a. Time responses at 30 seconds to a minute (or have no limit for deeper sharing).
   b. Put hands behind the back after responding to ensure a new person each time.
   c. End the activity without requiring everyone to have a turn, or ensure that each student gets one catch and response (e.g., during early community building). If using the former option, monitor participation and consider who may not be having a voice in class.
   d. Use two balls once comfort is reached using one. The second ball provides think time for one student while another is responding.
4. *Debrief* (2 minutes, optional): Begin with the default debrief questions (see p. 16) and see where the dialogue goes, or add the following prompts:
   a. How do you feel participating in play-based activities? Do you have any other forms of play in your life? How do you balance play and other activities?

b. How do you feel about deeper questions or hearing others share more deeply?
5. *Safety*: Minimal trust to use a throwable object is the baseline requirement for this activity. Beyond that, the trust requirement is flexible depending on the challenge level of the questions (see table 3.3). Some students may have challenges throwing or catching in which case the ball can be rolled on the floor (if students are in a circle), or simply carried from person to person. Partially deflating the ball makes for an easier, more inclusive activity. Questions that require a high degree of trust can be color-coded to give students a visual cue about a prompt's risk level.
6. *Integration Strategy*: Typically thumballs are used as a "get-to-know" or icebreaker activity but they can also have curriculum-related questions written on them. Using a numbered ball greatly facilitates changing questions for varying curriculum purposes, although, in most curriculum areas, a generic prompt can work well to
   a. activate prior knowledge at the start of a learning cycle;
   b. engage in critical thinking during learning via topic-of-the-week discussions; and/or
   c. review near the end of a learning cycle.

Keywords: choice, circle, empower, get-to-know, icebreaker, identity, integration, physical, social, short-'n'-safe

Table 3.3. Thumball Questions

Community Building and Get-To-Know	Curriculum and Learning
(The questions from the "low trust required" category of table 3.1 are ideal for a thumball.)	• One thing about [TOPIC] is . . . • A question I have about [TOPIC] is . . . • Regarding [TOPIC], I wonder . . . • One aspect of [TOPIC] I can explain . . . • One definition from [TOPIC] is . . . • [TOPIC], in my own words . . . • A key skill with [TOPIC] is . . . • If [TOPIC] is the answer, the question is . . . • I can connect [TOPIC] to . . . • An important thing about [TOPIC] is . . . • [TOPIC] is meaningful because . . .

SUPPLEMENTARIES: SHORT, SIMPLE, SAFE, OR SEARCHABLE SOCIAL WELL-BEING

- *Backchannels and Polls* are online services allowing students and teachers to share resources, participate in surveys or ask questions all using their own technology. Ideally, find a system that is free, does not require student personal information, and allows for moderation and voting of posts. *Search terms*: backchannel, classroom, polls.
- *Collaborative Group Skills* [Integration Strategy] takes advantage of the group work already happening in most classrooms to build priceless social skills. Prosocial group tasks must be truly collaborative and not just a way to split up work. Teachers also need to take time to *name, teach,* and *reflect* on group skills. These include self-regulation, participation, deep listening, time management, and building on the ideas of others. *Search terms*: group skills, collaborative, cooperative, group, learning.
- *Inside/Outside Circles* make connections rapidly using an inside circle facing outward and an outside circle facing in. Students spend a minute or less with the person across from them responding to get-to-know-you prompts (see p. 62) or curriculum questions. Rotates the circles in different ways to create new partners.
- *Interacting 1:1* is something we can forget to do in the busyness and business of school. Notice your balance of 1:1 interaction with students versus interacting with the whole class to discern if committing to some personal connections might be a good shift.
- *Media Ain't Social* challenges students to take a social media vacation for a day, week, or month. This involves restricting usage to ten minutes per day (or less), per platform to discover the benefits of in-person relationships. Millennials are the loneliest generation, with 38 percent often or always feeling lonely, compared to 23 percent of Generation X and 18 percent of Boomers.[24] But young students who reduced their social media use also reduced their loneliness, depression, and anxiety.[25] Invite students to use the found time to connect with others instead and debrief to explore any changes noticed from the vacation.

- *Mindful Dialogue* is a structured way to converse that deepens partner sharing on any curriculum or wellness topic. The teacher can model each stage shown below with a volunteer, with the ultimate intent that students will practice more uninterrupted listening, pausing, and paraphrasing on their own.
  1. Person A shares to B about the topic at hand (one minute). Pause.
  2. Person B paraphrases back to person A what they heard, and asks, "Is that it?"
  3. Person A confirms they got it (go to 4) or clarifies what was missed (go to 2).
  4. Reverse roles so person B shares to A, with paraphrasing by A.
- *Speakeasy Jigsaw* helps students understand different communication styles including assertive, aggressive, passive, passive-aggressive, manipulative, and more. Break the class in four to six groups, assigning a style to each group to research. The groups report back to the class (or a home group, see *jigsaw* p. 214), including a sample dialogue they have written using that style. Discuss when a particular style such as assertive, might be appropriate. *Search terms*: communication, styles, assertive, passive, aggressive.
- *The Three Filters* are a simple check that any communication—whether spoken, posted online, or sent electronically—is *true*, *necessary*, and *kind*. Write the filters on the board and make connections over time with comments made in class or online content. Talk about previewing messages, hitting send when upset, and how the three filters can help.
- *Visible Random Groups* are more agreeable, engaging, and prosocial than teacher-made or student-chosen groups.[26] Playing cards or free websites can make random, visible group-making easy and fun. *Search terms*: random, group.
- *Wishing Well* is a promise to silently say to each person you see, "I wish for you to be happy" followed by a personal wish: "I wish happiness for myself." Repeat throughout the day, making each connection a practice of kindness and self-compassion.

4

EUDAIMONIA

Meaning, Excellence, Growth, and Authenticity

"Things don't have purposes, as if the universe were a machine, where every part has a useful function. What's the function of a galaxy? I don't know if our life has a purpose and I don't see that it matters. What does matter is that we're a part. Like a thread in a cloth or a grass-blade in a field. It is and we are. What we do is like wind blowing on the grass."[1]

—Ursula K. Le Guin

What's the purpose of *your* life, or does being a part of life matter? More than 80 percent of American adults can answer these questions.[2] And most of these adults seek meaning regularly.[3] It's a different story with today's youth. One in three fifteen-year-olds feel their life has no clear meaning.[4] Is there a youth crisis of meaning, or is uncertainty just a natural part of growing up?

The teen years are synonymous with pleasure seeking but can also be a painful crucible where identity and purpose are deeply questioned. Wellness for many students is about having good times, or maybe getting to the gym. But these same teens might be surprised that this challenging phase of maturation is also a deeply sustaining source of *eudaimonic well-being*. Pleasure seeking (hedonia) has both positive and negative outcomes. But the eudaimonic domain of well-being is consistently positive for youth and even offsets some of the negatives.[5]

Eudaimonia is a delicious stew of self-discovery ingredients from the realm of positive psychology that combine to produce "MEGA" well-being.[6]

- **M**eaning in terms of coherence, purpose, significance, and a long-term view beyond self.
- **E**xcellence by applying signature strengths and virtue to reach a high standard.
- **G**rowth and self-discovery to develop full potential or self-actualization.
- **A**uthenticity through autonomy and personal expressiveness of an evolving identity.

Classroom sources of eudaimonia could be learning or teaching a beloved subject, hard-won achievement, or finding a life path that resonates strongly. These eudaimonic mega-vitamins are rich sources of thriving in their own right, but they also mutually reinforce each other, as well as other domains of wellness. Eudaimonia produces happiness, hope, positive relationships, and even longevity for students.[7] Teachers also have much to gain in this domain.

Joyce was three years from retirement as a high school English teacher. She had always been curious about new approaches but felt unmotivated after reading the last batch of essays. She signed up to audit a demonstration class at a neighboring high school and felt a stir in her chest when she walked in to see an open circle of students sitting in silent meditation. As the class unfolded, the authenticity of the teens' sharing moved Joyce deeply.

Afterward the demonstration class teacher said she had taken a mindfulness certification for educators and was part of a district pilot in social-emotional learning. At these words, Joyce felt a lightning bolt run up her spine. These experiences felt more meaningful than most essay topics she had ever assigned. Though she knew almost nothing about them, or how they would fit with the English curriculum, Joyce had a focus for her professional growth, even in the twilight of her career. She felt alive and energized, like she did in her first year of teaching.

It's never too late to discover, and strive toward, personally meaningful passions. But that's no reason to delay the eudaimonic search until after school. Grade 7–12 students can get a first taste of MEGA through academic counseling, career planning, or experiential learning programs already available in schools. Interest and aptitude surveys, digital portfolios, or the activities in this chapter add more ways to explore life pathways toward self-actualization.

AFFIRMING GENERATIONS

Before a student can even begin to think about authentic excellence, the benefit of expressing their truest self must outweigh the pain of hiding it. Michelle started her male to female transition in her third year of high school, and she was now in her senior year. Family and friends were supportive; however, some teachers still used he/his pronouns and even called her Seth. She'd been punched in the boys' bathroom or heard "What's he doing in here?" in the girls'. Michelle learned to hold it in every day, all day, in more ways than one.

Inclusive, affirming classrooms and schools are critical for cultivating eudaimonic well-being but are also just a beginning. Teachers must also actively challenge behaviors and beliefs that perpetuate bias. Allyship is a part, but author and journalist Ta-Nehisi Coates invites a collective stance: "I think one has to even abandon the phrase 'ally' and understand that you are not helping someone in a particular struggle; the fight is yours." We will struggle to walk our unique paths, no matter how meaningful, if it is painful or unsafe for anyone else to do so.

Establishing this groundwork to support eudaimonia is a priceless gift for youth, but it also offers an incredible reciprocity for teachers. Whatever their salary may be, one of a teacher's most precious benefits is the meaning derived from shaping young minds, hearts, and futures.

Research into the roots of eudaimonia show its strongest predictor is this very *generativity*: guiding, nurturing, and caring for the next generation.[8] Teachers who embrace the self-transcendent duty to foster young lives that extend beyond their own not only create a precious legacy but also enjoy a rare eudaimonic benefit few other careers provide.

Generativity is one source of meaning out of many that reveal the connections between eudaimonia and other domains. Transcendence of self through kindness to others and social connections (such as "Seeing and Sharing the Goodness," p. 78) boosts meaning and well-being, as does having a rich spiritual life. Having multiple sources of meaning increases wellness optimally, and buffers against the potential loss of any one source.[9] These sources are explored in the activities and supplementaries of this and other domains.

All this goodness has a prerequisite: teachers who authentically express their best selves in teaching and strive to grow in areas meaningful to them. It's no different for students, since working along a path to meaning or excellence feels good for everyone, and it is the heart of eudaimonia. No one activity can do this for all, but teachers who highlight the MEGA aspects of eudaimonia, and are willing to begin a eudaimonic journey themselves, light the way.

Key Messages

- Eudaimonia involves MEGA wellness: meaning, excellence, growth, and authenticity.
- Eudaimonia can be a more deeply sustaining source of well-being than hedonia.
- Experiential and guidance-related district programs may support eudaimonia.
- Actively countering barriers and bias helps students be and express their authentic selves.
- Teachers derive eudaimonic well-being from generativity: nurturing future generations.

EUDAIMONIC WELL-BEING ACTIVITIES

A Question of Purpose (Main Move)

"Ultimately, man should not ask what the meaning of his life is, but rather must recognize that it is he who is asked. In a word, each man is questioned by life; and he can only answer to life by answering for his own life; to life he can only respond by being responsible."[10]

—Viktor Frankl

"Why are we doing this?" is a question few teachers want to hear. And telling students the many wondrous purposes of your curriculum might not help, because—brace yourself—some of them just don't care about what you are teaching. This doesn't mean they don't like you or that the subject isn't inherently meaningful, it's just not meaningful for *them*. So if you feel passion for your subject, can you let that passion inspire them to find their own? And if you have answered some of your own "why" questions, can you invite them to answer theirs?

These answers don't come easily, for there is no rapid road to eudaimonia. Growth and excellence in the pursuit of authentic meaning is a lifelong, and uniquely individual, journey. But having something purposeful to live for is its own ongoing reward of wellness. When life has little meaning, it tends to feel unfulfilling no matter its ups and downs.[11] Many students, and some teachers, may be unaware of eudaimonia, or not have a clear sense of their purpose.

Wherever each road leads, a start can be had by unpacking the eudaimonic questions in this activity. The simple act of asking "What is my purpose?" can begin a quest for meaning. In the classroom context, supportive peers and teachers can help each other see their best strengths and share what eudaimonia means to them, perhaps inspiring others to find their own eureka moments. Pick up these questions, turn them over, work them, and let them do their work on you. Explore what it means to have a deeply sustaining life, fully lived. Can you help your students do the same? Can you help them find deep, personal, meaning?

Summary: Explore questions of what is meaningful and authentic personally.
Time: 5–15 minutes x four days
Trust Required: Medium

1. *Prep* (2–5 minutes): Teachers can make a copy of handout 4.1 "Questions of Purpose" for each student, or it may be best projecting them for everyone.
2. *Body Scan* (1 minute): Invite the class to close their eyes and do an inner body scan (see p. 149) for a minute. Sensitivity to inner feelings may help in the next step.

3. *Question Scan* (3 minutes): Refer students to the questions, inviting them to scan them in silence and write down question numbers that stand out for them, *without answering them*. With certain questions, they might feel a mental connection, body sensation, or inner spark, or just pick some. There is no "right" number of questions to pick: even one could be illuminating, where ten might not be. Students can focus on one question category or take a question from each. Emphasize that it's okay to not know any answers—that is expected. Finding at least one question to explore is great.
4. *Reflecting and Exploring* (5–10 minutes × 3+ days): Students reflect on their chosen questions over several days or even weeks, writing responses and notes. They may not have answers at first, but the point is to openly explore the questions: take them home, sleep on them, and ask close friends, family, or caring adults for their thoughts. Spend 5–10 minutes pairing them with different partners to discuss their responses, and eliciting some whole class sharing. Doing the activity yourself as a teacher allows you to contribute meaningfully to the discussion and perhaps inspire students in some way.
5. *Circle Debrief* (20 minutes): This activity may activate significant thoughts and feelings around meaning. Approach this circle debrief as sacred, and make this sacredness clear to the class (see p. 62). Resurface agreements and use a talking piece to ensure deep listening and sharing. Invite students to share what stood out for them in the questions and their responses. Use a non-sequential approach (p. 61) to take pressure off anyone who does not wish to share. Let authenticity and meaning be the focus of the circle, and see what that meaning does for the entire group, including the teacher.
6. *Safety*: Some students may have some difficulty with interoception (see p. 22). Others may have had prior experiences that made expressing authentic identity unsafe. Others may

realize their lives don't line up with what is truly meaningful to them, and that can also be unsettling. Time and support can bring self-care and equanimity, so split up the activity over multiple days to give students a chance to seek the support if needed.
7. *Integration Strategy*: While a student may find some aspect of the curriculum to be meaningful, most will find meaning in another path. Whatever subject you teach, helping a young person find their path might be the greatest learning you could ever provide.
8. *Lifeplay*: The ultimate lifeplay invitation is to pursue these answers, or keep asking the questions, as purpose and eudaimonia are lifelong pursuits. Can students get out there and see how they can make their meaning real? Can they volunteer, learn, and launch themselves along their own path of purpose and significance? What can they do in the next two weeks to take the next step (see MEGA-SMARTER Goal Journeys, p. 100)?

Keywords: card, caring, circle, choice, empower, eudaimonia, foundational, get-to-know, identity, lifeplay, mindfulness

---

Handout 4.1. Questions of Purpose

Name: _____

These questions can help explore what meaning, excellence, growth, and authenticity mean to you personally. Scan these questions, writing down or circling the question numbers that stand out for you, without answering them. Notice which questions give you a sensation in your body or a mental spark. There is no "right" number of questions to pick: even one could be illuminating. It's okay to have a feeling of not having answers—that is expected.

Table 4.1. Questions of Purpose

Category	Question
Questions of Doing	1. What do you do, or want to do, that feels important or meaningful to you?
	2. Is there anything that you deeply enjoy or that gives you a sense of accomplishment, even if you don't succeed much or at all?
	3. What activities make you feel alive, fuel your passion, or make the most satisfying use of your time?
	4. Have you ever felt so engaged in an energizing flow, such that time passed unnoticed or you even forgot to eat?
	5. Is there something you deeply enjoyed or appreciated when you were younger, even if you don't do it now?
Questions of Dreaming	6. What directions in life feel most important or significant for you?
	7. What do you truly want of this world, and what is the world wanting of you?
	8. If money, or the expectations of others, weren't an issue, what then?
Questions of Feeling	9. Is there a feeling, energy, or vibe inside you (which may be hard to put into words) that is important or powerful for you?
	10. Have you ever had an experience when you felt absolute bliss, connection, empowerment, freedom, tranquility, or something similarly powerful?
	11. What was your essential nature when you were young, or what did you experience purely and authentically when you were young?
	12. When have you felt most like "you"?
Questions of Growing	13. Is there a form of personal growth or development that appeals to you deeply, or where perfecting your skills feels awesome?
	14. What are your best qualities and skills?
	15. What strengths or qualities do friends or classmates see in you (ask them)?

Category	Question
Questions of Loving	16. Who are the most important people in your life?
	17. What kinds of relationships or social situations inspire you, fire you up, or feel the most meaningful to you?
Questions of Opposing	18. Are you putting off anything important (perhaps for fear of failure or judgment, or to please others in some way)?
	19. Have you ever felt like you "weren't yourself"? What is the opposite of that?
	20. Is there something others struggle with that you actually like?
	21. Is there anything you are currently pursuing that isn't working for you, which you could let go of, to focus on your highest calling?
Questions of Transcending	22. Does caring for others, or the world beyond you, inspire you in some way?
	23. Does connecting to the unlimited, beyond the self (whatever that means for you) inspire you in some way?
	24. Is there a cause, ideal, or issue that you feel is deeply important to you and for which you want to make an impact?
	25. What are the most important values to you? Can you prioritize your top five, three, or one?

Inviting Identity: Creating Classroom Spaces that Support Authentic Self-Expression

"We need people to stand up and take on the problems borne of oppression as their own, without remove or distance. We need people to do this even if they cannot fully understand what it's like to be oppressed for their race or ethnicity, gender, sexuality, ability, class, religion, or other marker of identity. We need people to use common sense to figure out how to participate in social justice."[12]

—Roxane Gay

For some students, repressing their true identity is a painful norm. Expressing one's true self—being vulnerable—can hurt more than diminishing oneself or even pretending to be someone else. Many students are not showing who they are fully out of fear of being judged, bullied, or getting in trouble. But hiding vital aspects of identity inhibits well-being immensely. That's why teachers who have the courage and compassion to create safer and inclusive classroom spaces offer a significant eudaimonic gift.

Whatever identities a teacher may have, they also have power. In classical physics, power is a transfer of energy over time. Teachers can create safer spaces by shifting energy, over time, to those who don't have as much privilege or power. This could mean giving the spotlight, the microphone, or extra resources to students who need them to find success or self-express. It takes humility to not take the comfortable center in the classroom, instead putting those who have never been there a little closer. In this way, inequality can be the road to equity.

This section offers four different activities, along a continuum of trust required, to provide entry points for self-expression. While there's no guarantee that students will want to (or be able to) open up, a great deal can be done to make any opening more welcoming. The following list of teacher considerations, preparations, and actions are essential "prep" components to that welcoming, and for these activities in general.

Teacher Considerations

- Discovering and expressing one's authentic self is a major source of eudaimonic well-being; hiding and repressing it is a major source of harm.
- Identity is multifaceted and fluid, resulting in multiple, beautiful layers of expression that can change over time.
- Each person decides for themselves who they are and what they will share. Pressuring students to share in any activity could cause harm.
- Multiple, complex forms of oppression exist in every classroom.
- It's the work of all teachers to understand, talk about, and remove these barriers.

- In safer classrooms, power flows from those who have privilege to those who lack it.
- Authentic sharing is correlated to the depth of safety, freedom, and love in the classroom.

Teacher Preparations

- Know yourself: your identities, beliefs, social position, your privileges, and areas where you experience a lack of privilege. Deeply examine yourself for the inevitable gaps in knowledge, and implicit biases, that are impacting everything you do, from the materials you choose, to the ways you teach, to how you respond to students.
- Know your learners: teachers alone are responsible for enlarging their understanding of historic and current oppression, and the strengths and lives of their students today.
- Build healthy student-teacher and student-student relationships (see social well-being, p. 55) as a foundation for exploring identity.
- Cultivate emotional skills, such as understanding and regulating feelings (see emotional well-being, p. 175), as a support for safer and deeper eudaimonic work.
- Make it clear to students through your words, actions, and being that creating a safer, caring space is a priority.
- Choose and use classroom resources that affirm a spectrum of diverse identities. Seek to understand what resonates with students by listening to them, and ensure that each student can see that their life is expressed in classroom life, over time.
- Continuously seek the perspectives of students, particularly the underrepresented, to guide learning and well-being work, both overtly and also through anonymous feedback.

Teacher Actions

- Address harmful language or actions immediately—as they arise—no matter who is present, taking decisive and public action.
- Allow students to share what they wish to share—no more, no less.
- Affirm and allow for multiple layers of identities to emerge and change over time.

- Find ways to empower student strengths and voices in the classroom.
- Connect with students' communities, including families and community. Seek, reflect on, and respond to anonymous feedback (p. 40). Notice if students are engaging deeply, or hiding and playing along, and adjust accordingly.
- When you mess up, apologize, and ask how to make things better.
- Adapt activities to provide more safety or anonymity where needed.
- Participate as a teacher, affirming your own identity and validating self-expression.

Digging in with students is key to both student and teacher well-being: sharing all the beautiful parts of oneself. Working at this depth with students may feel daunting, but it's possible for any teacher and class to make progress, wherever they may begin. Cultivating a safe space to explore authentic identity rewards both students and teachers through:

- personal self-reflection and consideration of one's truest self;
- vulnerable interpersonal sharing leading to lasting connections to self and others;
- powerful emergence, expression, and evolution of authentic identity;
- transformative healing, learning, and growth in a safe and loving classroom.

Summary: Choose from four activities that invite students to share about themselves.
Time: Varies
Trust Required: Varies

1. *We Wall* (low trust, 30 minutes): Give students cardstock that they fold in half to create a card. On the outside of the card, students are invited to put images that represent who they are, what matters to them, or information about themselves such as hobbies, favorite snacks, or things about their family. Inside, they write their name, and paste a photo or any image

that represents who they are. Post these around the room, then invite students to circulate silently and learn about their classmates, and what matters to them, inside and out.[13]

2. *Story of My Life* (low to medium trust, 40 minutes): Students use any one of the following prompts to write about themselves, either for self-reflection (low trust) or *optional* sharing (medium trust). Students must never feel pressured to share; in safer spaces, they will share deeply, resulting in powerful autonomy and authenticity.
    a. "If somebody wrote the story of your life, what would they need to include?"
    b. "Write an autobiography that explores who you are as a learner and how past experiences have shaped your sense of self."
    c. "If you look back on the person you were four years ago, what advice would you give yourself?"
    d. "Can you describe a few characteristics of yourself four years ago and a few that describe you now? What has changed—and why?"

3. *About My Name* (medium to high trust, 25 minutes): Students explore how their names, and the story of their names, has reflected and shaped their identity. The following prompts could be used in a circle discussion to elicit non-sequential (that is, optional) responses from students, with the teacher also sharing first in a genuine way. Some students may not be ready, willing, or able, to talk about their name (or any identity) for any number of reasons. This a high-trust activity, appropriate when significant classroom community, trust, and safety has been established.
    a. "Can you tell a story about your name? Where does your name come from? What does your name mean to you?"
    b. "Do different people have different names, or nicknames, for you? Are those names of your choosing?"
    c. "How do you want to be addressed?

4. *A Portrait of Identities* (high trust): Students explore aspects of their identity privately, for self-reflection. Make all sharing in this activity *very* optional. Aspects of identity can include any or all of faith, gender identity or expression, history, origin (national or ethnic), physical ability, race, sexual orientation, and socioeconomic status. It's critical for students to explore the intersections of these aspects as well (e.g., being gender fluid and biracial). As with any activity, teachers participate themselves. Consider using one of the following approaches to create and explore this portrait of authentic self.
    a. Give students a blank sheet on which to draw their identity as a sketch, word cloud, or overlapping circles of identity—however they wish. The teacher could then present a list of aspects of identity (see list above, or a human rights code) and tell students, "Think about the ways you express your identity or the ways you see yourself. Pick the ones that you really think about most often."
        i. Students can then continue to explore, and self-reflect, on their identity.
        ii. Affirming identities throughout the year may result in changes.
    b. Ask students to focus on one, two, or a few aspects or intersections:
        i. where they feel a sense of belonging or privilege;
        ii. where they feel they are hiding or excluded;
        iii. which feel most important or central to who they are; and/or
        iv. which they feel others understand the least.
5. *Debrief* (x minutes): The debrief below is applicable to any of the above options, though student sharing, especially for higher trust activities, is optional. Teacher qualities (see p. 35) of sensitivity, vulnerability, and compassion are essential in such discussions. It may be appropriate to not debrief as

a class. Instead, journal, talk to students privately, or refer those who need support. Gauging the safety in the room (p. 50), and using the considerations, preparations and actions above will guide decisions about debriefing. The standard debrief questions (p. 16) are a start, and then the following prompts could be explored:
   a. What have you learned about yourself? What have you learned about others?
   b. Are there parts that others don't understand or misinterpret about you?
   c. What's one thing you would want to share about yourself?
   d. Is it easier to be your authentic self or pretend to be something else in school?
   e. What surprised you about yourself or others?
6. *Safety*: Review one more time the considerations, preparations, and actions listed above.
7. *Lifeplay*: Students can be encouraged to continue the reflection at home, with their families and in their communities, fostering more dialogue and shared understanding of each person's unique identity.
8. *Integration Strategy*: Most curriculum documents have a lot to say about equity, inclusion, or human rights, often including an entire section on the topic. See how these documents guide teachers in finding curricular applications and touchstones for including equity work as part of well-being.

Keywords: caring, circle, choice, emotional, empower, eudaimonia, get-to-know, identity, integration, journal, lifeplay, safety, schoolwide, social, support

MEGA-SMARTER Goal Journeys

> "You need to pivot away from what's worked for others and toward what works for you. Have your own "Eureka!" moments. Discover for yourself what rouses genuine and heartfelt positivity."[14]
>
> —Barbara Fredrickson

Growth and excellence are at the core of eudaimonia, but what feels authentic to a particular student may not match the status quo. Passing the piano exam, landing a part-time job, or getting into that school Mom and Mum went all sound great, but are any of these genuine for the student? The excellence and growth aspects of eudaimonia activate fully with goals that feel authentically worthwhile. When a meaningful purpose can be articulated, and efforts aligned to that purpose, the result can be a resonant life of meaning that produces abundant well-being.

Striving for a goal that stirs the heart, provides a deep and lasting satisfaction even where there is a failure to achieve it. On the other hand, pursuing uninspiring goals can be drudgery, and attaining even fame or fortune might only give fleeting satisfaction. Eudaimonic pursuits are clearly more strongly tied to wellness than pleasure-seeking, and their effects last longer.[15]

Consider Gregor Mendel, the founder of modern genetics. His monumental research on genetic inheritance was ignored by the scientific community, and he faced social barriers from a life of poverty as well as mental health challenges. He even failed (twice) to become a high school teacher and ended up being recognized for his achievements only decades after his death. But he clearly felt a eudaimonic well-being in the meaning of his work and his long-term view: "My scientific studies have afforded me great gratification; and I am convinced that it will not be long before the whole world acknowledges the results of my work."

This activity provides a template for eudaimonic goal-setting and a process for an entire class to pursue those goals, potentially activating every element of MEGA. Goals may be personal, but working at them as a class allows for group check-ins and accountability. As teachers and students move through their goal arcs together, they can support each other and even work together if aims align. What's critical is that it all means something: the journey is as rewarding as the achievement, and the entire process becomes a lasting source of wellness.

Summary: Collectively pursue meaningful goals together over the span of a course or unit.
Time: 60+ minutes (split up over a period of weeks or months)
Trust Required: Low

1. *Prep* (5 minutes): Prepare copies of handout 4.2 for students. Consider a time frame for this activity, which could be a few weeks—or even months (timings are all flexible).
2. *A Question of Purpose* (optional): Consider exploring this meaning-making activity first (p. 88), to help students discover meaningful goal directions. If goals are being set within a particular curricular area instead of a personal one, this step may be omitted.
3. *Goal Examples* (5 minutes): Brainstorm examples of MEGA-SMARTER goals, in addition to the environmental one on handout 4.2. Highlight the importance of *meaning* in each example, for this is what distinguishes typical goals from MEGA-goals.[16] Also be sure to point out whether the examples have SMARTER aspects or not. More examples follow:
    a. "I will apply for three summer jobs or internships, one per week: with the animal hospital, with an animal researcher, and with the humane society." [Goal for a student who loves animals, and feels joy being around them.]
    b. "I will write 2,000 words per week for three weeks to complete at least one chapter of my first novel." [A teacher who has always wanted to write, and loves being in the flow of writing, but has not written in years.]
    c. [Also see "Scaffolding Alternatives" below for more ideas.]
4. *Goal Crafting* (20 minutes, split over multiple sessions): Students use handout 4.2 to craft and draft a meaningful goal statement. Give an end date, though goals may stretch beyond it. Elicit some sharing (and share personally as the teacher) to clarify the MEGA-SMARTER criteria. Take a few days to do this, and let students know that crafting a meaningful goal is a challenging achievement on its own.
5. *Safety*: Review student goals and inform caregivers of the project to support students.

6. *Scaffolding Options*: If goal setting does not resonate, or seems complex, students can explore these alternatives, all of which are fertile eudaimonic ground (if not goals per se):
   - Volunteering in a way that feels personally meaningful
   - Contributing to—or especially fighting for—a personally significant cause
   - Deepening connections with people who personally matter
   - Learning and growing in a personally meaningful area
   - Expressing gratitude and appreciation (see p. 199), especially to other people
   - Writing personal values, repeating them daily, and standing by them
7. *Goal Striving Lifeplay* (several weeks or months): Students and teacher work toward their goals on their own as personal lifeplay. Let them know that with truly worthwhile goals, there will be well-being found in striving alone, and that the class will have several debriefs during the process. Get excited; this could lead to something big!
8. *Monitor and Debrief* (5 minutes x multiple times): Using any of the following options.
   a. Honestly share your personal teacher goal journey first to model for students.
   b. Students self-reflect on goal progress using the "TER" rows of the template. A lack of progress could be a lack of meaning, rather than effort. Meaningful, stretch goals require hard work, but that effort will feel rewarding, not chore-like.
   c. Pair up students with an accountability partner to share goal progress and experiences, and/or share as a class.
   d. Invite students to rework *any* aspect of a goal (see the following examples):
      i. M: deciding a goal isn't as *meaningful* as originally thought, and rework
      ii. T: adjusting *timing*, or finding someone else to help (*team*)

iii. R: consider how to address *roadblocks* and adapt to them
   e. Debrief using the standard questions, especially focusing on *impact* and *change*.
   f. Celebrate efforts made, progress or not. Goal setting and achieving are major eudaimonic skills that take time to develop.
9. *Integration Strategy*: Any curriculum-based project significant enough to be broken into goal steps could be a basis for this activity. Passion projects are a wonderful fit, since students have freedom to choose personally meaningful topics within a curricular area.
10. *Schoolwide Extension*: Use this process with any school team, club, or group to set personal or group goals, bringing even more meaning to co-curriculars.

Keywords: caring, choice, creative, empower, eudaimonia, integration, lifeplay, schoolwide

---

Handout 4.2. MEGA-SMARTER Goal Journeys

Name: _____

Meaning, excellence, growth, and authenticity (MEGA) are the core of eudaimonic well-being. Use this MEGA-SMARTER goal template to develop a goal that is personally meaningful and powerful, and then pursue that goal until _____ (teacher-provided end date).

Example: "For three weeks, I will research five different environmental groups per week (at least one of which will be local), to see which are most engaging to me. The research will include visiting websites, making notes, and reaching out with an inquiry about how I could work with them. By March 31, I will have decided which one to support and would have begun volunteering." [Goal set by a student who is an environmental champion.]

The workspace below will help you develop your own meaningful goal, and then track it in the coming weeks and months as you work toward it. Be prepared to share progress with classmates periodically. Feel free to review and adjust any aspect of your goal at any time. While your goal may benefit others, it is truly *yours*, so reflect deeply on what is most meaningful for *you*.

Table 4.2. **MEGA-SMARTER Goals**

	Traditional Goal Considerations	*MEGA Goal Considerations*	*Goal Workspace*
S	Can you write a **specific** and **simple** goal statement that anyone could understand?	Is this goal so **significant** to you, that working toward it might feel as good as achieving it?	
M	Is the goal **measurable** in some way, so you can know how you are doing?	Is this goal **meaningful** to achieve, and perhaps goes beyond benefitting you personally?	
A	Is this goal **achievable** (not too easy or boring, but not too hard so as to cause anxiety). Is it pitched to challenge you just right?	Is this goal **authentic** for you, rather than what others want for you? Consider this deeply.	
R	Is this goal **realistic** and do you have the **resources** you need to achieve it? If needed, break your goal into smaller steps.	Is this goal **relevant** to you, and your life's purpose?	
T	Is there a **time-frame** for this goal? Include dates, and what will be achieved at each step.	Can you connect with a **team** of people which can support you in this goal?	

	Traditional Goal Considerations	MEGA Goal Considerations	Goal Workspace
E	How will you **evaluate** your progress?	**Enjoy** by celebrating each effort, milestone (and even failure) along the way. Well-being is in the journey itself, not just the ends.	
R	Will **readjusting** any aspect of this journey serve my highest purpose better?	What **roadblocks** might be (or is being) encountered? How will I address it?	

Goal Statement:

Goal Notes:

Animal Groups: Schools of Thought

This game provides a context for the exploration of identity, inclusion, barriers to belonging, and othering. It also highlights the basic human need to feel connected to others and explores the balance of finding authentic autonomy in balance with belonging to groups. The game may be conducted with staff or students, and it works very well as a fishbowl (p. 190), where neutral observers may uncover subtle interactions.

> **Summary**: Simulate forming animal groups to explore identity, autonomy, and group dynamics.
> **Time**: 20 minutes
> **Trust Required**: High
>
> 1. *Prep* (5 minutes): Create animal cards by simply writing animal names on slips of paper or printing free online animal cards. Make multiples of most animals with at least two being unique; for example, 1 dog, 1 horse, 2 cats, 3 cows, 4 turkeys, 5 sheep, 6 chickens, and 8 ducks for a class of 30 students. Make space for free movement or get outside (p. 212).
> 2. *Explain* (1 minute): Distribute an animal identity to each student, which they keep secret. Invite them to simply "form groups without speaking." Don't say anything specific about how to form groups. Remind them not to speak, although sounds and gestures are okay.
> 3. *Grouping* (3 minutes): Observe students literally behaving like animals as they search and form groups. Watch for behaviors that may be debriefed, such as apprehension at not belonging to a group, or relief on finding one (see Mx. Pereira's story, p. 14). Notice if anyone hides their card or joins a non-matching group rather than being alone. Someone may proudly form a group of one. Anything could be a rich topic for discussion.

4. *Debriefing* (10 minutes): Pause the activity to debrief when magical teaching learning moments occur. Ask students about their choices and behaviors, inviting group discussion. Use the standard prompts (p. 16) as well as the deeper prompts below (optional). Sharing is optional, or it can be done anonymously with snowballs (p. 42) or an online note tool. Students may also reflect privately and then share at their option.
   a. What assumptions were made about group forming?
   b. How do we tend to make groups in the real world?
   c. What is the impact of feeling like we belong, or not, to a group?
   d. How does grouping lead to othering?
   e. Why do we make groups at all?
   f. How can self-acceptance support belonging (see Brené Brown, p. 56)?
   g. Can true belonging include not being part of any group?
   h. Is it easier to be yourself, or someone else, at school?
   i. Is there anywhere you can be your truest self?
5. *Safety*: This is a high-trust activity requiring significant classroom courage and community. Due to systemic oppression in our schools and society, some students will already feel excluded from their peers due to their identities. Knowing this, be sure you have a foundational understanding of systemic oppression and have created an inclusive classroom. Most cards are distributed randomly, but the solo cards could be given intentionally to confident students who have strong social positionality.

Keywords: caring, collaborative, emotional, eudaimonia, hedonia, identity, outdoors, social

SUPPLEMENTARIES: SHORT, SIMPLE, SAFE, OR SEARCHABLE EUDAIMONIC WELL-BEING

- *Altruism* is a classic eudaimonic vector, so make it a classroom discussion topic over a period of months, giving students time to engage in some informal giving, goodwill, or even volunteering, while debriefing the impact on self and others.
- *Best Self* is a potential-realizing writing task or journal entry where students describe their best qualities and proudest moments.[17] Virtues vocab (p. 31) can spark some starting points, and sharing (always optional) can provide social elevation (p. 66).
- *Class Talking Piece* invites everyone in the classroom to add a quotation (written on a tag), favorite word, signature or other personal touch to a stone, stick, plush toy, or other object. This piece then becomes a sacred talking piece for use with circles.
- *Celebrating Growth and Excellence* is baked into school culture with formal reporting and the usual awards, but anecdotal or verbal praise also provides eudaimonic wellness. Teachers can send informal notes home or recognize students publicly in class. Students typically underrepresented in traditional success structures (especially academics) can benefit from being recognized meaningfully in these ways. Explicit acknowledgment of student self-discovery or reaching potential (beyond the usual math tests and essay writing) can be especially consequential. While evaluation of growth is typically in the teacher's purview, sharing power with students (by encouraging them to notice and celebrate others as per "Catching Goodness," p. 66) is incredible for self-actualization.
- *Digital Portfolios* help students recognize the best in themselves by curating and displaying that which best reflects their personal MEGA qualities. A variety of free, online portfolio tools are available. All of them allow sharing (with peers, teachers, family, and community) for feedback, metacognitive self-reflection, and celebration. Portfolios help students reflect on personal growth and take ownership of their success, for a host of educational and eudaimonic benefits. *Search terms*: digital, student, portfolios.
- *Hobby Talk* explores the things students and teachers do that are genuinely and intrinsically rewarding (love to do), rather than an

extrinsic goal or responsibility (have to do). Talking about hobbies, whether as part of a circle or a short discussion at the end of a period, builds understanding and connections around similar interests. Get some extra elevation by asking what it is that sparks love, joy, or meaning from the hobby.
- *I am . . . I am not . . .* are two identity-defining (and denying) prompts to which students (and teacher) can respond again and again. Responses could be journal entries, or written responses using a page of copied "I am . . . " and "I am nots . . . " or a voluntary circle round, with each student giving an "I am . . . " or "I am not . . . " statement that can be repeated as many times as is fruitful.
- *The Ladder of Student Participation* is a framework for student empowerment developed by Roger Hart, presenting a continuum from manipulation to shared decision making.[18] Use the ladder with other staff to consider ways to involve students more deeply in all aspects of classroom or school life such as classroom routines, events, committees, teams, and more. The ladder is not meant to be hierarchical, or absolute, yet provides a way to think about student autonomy, a key facet of eudaimonia. *Search terms*: ladder, student, involvement, classroom, passion, project.
- *Love Letter to Self* involves writing a self-compassionate love letter to yourself. Give students high-quality paper and invite them to write at the beginning of a learning cycle, then read them and self-reflect near the end of the cycle. Teachers participate fully.
- *Mapping Me* uses free, online mind-mapping tools, or pen and paper, to draw a mind map representing and celebrating self: interests, skills, goals, achievements, and (most importantly), what is personally meaningful. *Search terms*: mind-mapping, classroom.
- *More Than One Story* is a free, online bank of questions for small-group circles that facilitates empathy, inclusion, and understanding as participants share personal stories.[19] One person (usually the teacher) begins by responding to a question prompt and telling a story. Others can ask follow-up questions, until the storyteller is done, at which point the next person can have a turn. *Search terms*: more than one story.
- *Student Choice and Voice* shares classroom power by giving students input, choice, or outright design control over learning topics,

classroom resources, assignments, tasks, test questions, and assessment criteria. *Search terms*: student, choice.
- *Student Self-Assessment* is an underrated approach to assessment with potential for MEGA eudaimonia. Students involved in their own assessment better understand success criteria, leading to self-actualization and internal motivation, not to mention better achievement. The higher-order thinking of grade 7–12 students makes subjective assessment possible (see options below). *Search terms*: student self-assessment.
    - Students reflecting on their own learning skills and study habits
    - Students comparing an assignment in progress against a rubric to self-adjust
    - Students developing the assessment criteria for a checklist or rubric
    - Students taking up, and marking, their own quizzes or tests. (Give students a weird-colored crayon given to do it, coach them in the mark scheme, and check everything afterward for accuracy as they learn to self-assess)
- *"That's Me!"* puts student names, stories, photos (or other aspects of student lives) into classroom materials and handouts in sensitive ways, boosting identity and engagement.
- *Unlabeling* is a discussion where students reflect on personal characteristics or labels that may have become reinforced, whether by themselves or others. Possible prompts include the following:
    - Consider which label(s) we may have been given, or given to ourselves: *athlete, caregiver, creator, explorer, helper, hero, innocent, intellectual, jester, lover, outlaw, performer, rebel, ruler, sage, spiritual, visionary*.
    - Respond to the prompt "I'm a [blank] person," thinking of the first word or two that comes to mind and discuss.
    - How do these labels serve, and how do they constrain?
    - Can we let go of labels, or make space for new ones? Can we be any label?

5

RESILIENCE

Transforming Challenge into Thriving

> "Of all the virtues we can learn, no trait is more useful, more essential for survival, and more likely to improve the quality of life than the ability to transform adversity into an enjoyable challenge."[1]
>
> —Mihaly Csikszentmihalyi

In 1906, Herbert Jennings observed single-celled, pond-dwelling ciliates adapting to contaminants (carmine powder) placed in their environment.[2] He made the remarkable discovery that even primitive forms of life could respond well to adversity—that they exhibited *resilience*. However, Jennings's findings were discredited in a 1967 study that detected supposed flaws in his work. Fifty-two years later (in a fittingly parallel display of scientific and unicellular resilience), a 2019 team of scientists used video microscopy to prove once again that this tiny, ancient form of life does indeed adapt to challenge in diverse ways.[3]

From single-celled organisms to the most complex forms of life, adversity is an unavoidable life experience, with resilience as its vital response. The inevitability of disappointment, difficulty, and even disaster make resilience a crucial trait for surviving and thriving. Yet as common as suffering may be, when it isn't shared with others, there may be a feeling of being alone. The truth is that others have challenges too, and with those same others we can access and develop resilience together.

The last day of the training series on restorative practices had been deeply transformative for the teacher participants, who came from schools all over the district. In a closing circle, each participant was asked to share the impact of the learning on them. This typically resulted in expressions of gratitude and good intentions for the classroom—but not this day. A solemn silence descended as the very first teacher shared that his mother was dying in a hospice. In visiting her each day, he could see a precious window of forgiveness opening between them.

The rawness of his words brought a few tears to the circle, and opened the heart of the next person, who spoke of living with ADHD as an adult and a teacher. What followed was a magical and powerful succession of revelations that unveiled a powerful truth: *everyone* has *something*. The circle left some in a state of wonder, others feeling empathy, others uplifted, but all with the sacred knowing that both suffering and resilience are universal.

Schools are fabulous incubators for resilience, providing many challenges and the social support to respond to them. Hard times may be an inevitability in classrooms, but they are also an opportunity and a possibility: an opportunity to boost life satisfaction and positive emotions;[4] a possibility for finding post-traumatic growth, meaning, and authenticity (key for eudaimonia); all while reducing emotional or behavioral problems.[5] For these reasons, explicitly developing resilience in youth is the vital work of schools.

While there are few curriculum standards for resilience, grit programs have surged in popularity. Yet grit differs from resilience and is more about sticking to goals rather than recovering from setbacks. For youth facing systemic barriers, a focus on grit can even be harmful.[6] Determination alone cannot overcome unjust racial bias, gender barriers, crippling poverty, or other forms of systemic oppression. Before a student thinks they must "grit out" bias, removing systemic barriers must be our collective moral priority. Activist and author bell hooks understood that "being oppressed means the absence of choices," highlighting this imperative.[7]

An implication of this is that resilience is more than overcoming difficulty. Adapting well is indeed a core resilience skill, but so too is the way difficulty itself is experienced. Wellness can be gleaned from difficulty (systemic barriers excluded) so that some forms of adversity do not have to be seen as purely problematic. Fortunately, these perspectives, and other resilience traits (see table 5.1), can be explored explicitly in class.[8]

When Eshe broke her collarbone in field hockey practice just six days before the playoffs, her coach had a fit, and her parents freaked. Eshe was the star player, there was no backup goalkeeper, and some scouts were scheduled to see her play. But somewhere on the drive to the hospital, in a brief moment of silence, Eshe had a clear intuition. The daily "thought of the day" on the announcements came back to her: *"Your peace about what is happening is proportional to your acceptance of what is happening."* Her body relaxed, and she felt relief wash over her. She knew that the way through today, and the weeks to come, would be total acceptance—of everything. She felt sad thinking about not playing with her team but also light as a feather.

TRAITS OF RESILIENCE

Eshe exemplified one of many traits of resilience, shown in table 5.1. Her resilience was not in adapting but in *accepting*. Resilience has many more facets than simply "dealing" with adversity. Jean Chatzky, author, journalist, and CEO, explains: "Resilience isn't a single skill. It's a variety of skills and coping mechanisms." Exploring this full spectrum of traits offers much to students and educators, especially those facing additional barriers, such as Indigenous or transgender people. Each trait below is developed through the activities in this chapter.

Connections with other wellness domains shine through these traits, making resilience multi-modal. Sources of resilience can be found across the entire spectrum of well-being:

- flow and self-directed neuroplasticity in cognitive well-being (p. 143)
- gratitude and optimism in emotional well-being (p. 175)
- finding support from trusted others in social well-being (p. 55)

- finding meaning and growth from struggle in eudaimonica (p. 85)
- stress and struggle as a doorway to spiritual experience (p. 235)

Table 5.1. Traits of Resilience

Category	Trait
Traits of Buffing (a gaming term) prepare for adversity ahead of time (think "equip heat shield to endure fire").	1. Cultivating awareness, intuition, emotional regulation, self-confidence, self-compassion, self-care, and flexibility. 2. Developing a network of caring and supportive others: friends, family, colleagues, and community members.
Traits of Reframing take a positive perspective, appreciating adversity and seeing it as necessary and even beneficial.	3. Being hopeful through an optimistic, realistic, long-term outlook, and not catastrophizing in the face of adversity. 4. Feeling grateful for the good things in life, from the contrast of experiencing the not-so-good. 5. Welcoming uncertainty and challenge as the nature of life.
Traits of Dealing are the traditional and vital skills of engaging with difficulty actively and effectively.	6. Focusing efforts in circles of control and influence. 7. Making wise, loving, skillful decisions in adversity. 8. Taking wise, loving, skillful actions in adversity. 9. Seeking immersive states in the midst of dealing.
Traits of Experiencing tap into the vibrancy and peace of experiencing difficulty exactly as it is.	10. Accepting (not resisting) that which cannot be changed to reduce subjective suffering. 11. Deeply feeling difficult moments fully, imbuing life with meaning and poignancy (not reframing or avoiding).
Traits of Growing derive learning and change from each setback, making us stronger with every challenge faced.	12. Thriving and changing after stress, difficulty, or loss. 13. Seeing and even *relishing* setbacks and adversity as not just indicators of growth, but the wrapper in which can be found nuggets of learning, love, and redemption. 14. Discovering new resilience traits and strengths in ourselves.

Teachers will benefit from these traits as much as students, both professionally and personally.

The rain picked up as Andrew wound his car through the lot, not too late to teach his first class, but not too early either. Students had taken most of the close spots, but he found a space at the end of the lot where the forest began. He pulled in and shut off the engine to pause for a few seconds, as was his habit. His senses began to stand out as his busy thoughts subsided.

The blue-green of the spruce trees smeared by the sheeting rain on the windshield reminded him of his troubles, and his heart broke open anew. The breakup wasn't recent, and yet he felt the whole of it in that moment, as fresh and painful as the day it happened. He let go in the car, sobbing at first, then keening, feeling at the end of the world. At the bottom, he felt a newfound clarity. A recognition that this was actually a priceless experience. He knew for the first time that the depth of this devastation was also the height of his love. He realized he didn't *have* to feel this; he *got* to feel this. Andrew stepped out into the rain, scoured but clear.

Whether for teachers or students, resilience is not just overcoming, but welcoming, appreciating, and flowing with the full breadth of human life. Classrooms are great places to explore this breadth, and the spectrum of resilience traits, for lasting well-being.

Key Messages

- Resilience has many traits beyond adapting or enduring including *buffing* (cultivating protective traits), *reframing* (optimism and appreciation for challenge), *dealing* (good decisions and actions in the face of adversity), *experiencing* (accepting and feeling difficulty fully), and *growing* (thriving and changing beyond hardship).
- Resilience is strongly supported and connected to other domains of well-being.

RESILIENCE ACTIVITIES

Response-Ability Part I: Choice Moments (Main Move)

> "Our current understanding of emotion lags far behind our understanding of nearly every other aspect of life. We can chart the universe and split the atom, but we can't seem to understand or manage our natural emotional reactions to provoking situations."[9]
>
> —Karla McLaren

Ruth had hustled to make it to class after the lunchtime science department meeting. She was giving lab instructions and the class had just settled in when Theo edged in late, again.

When Ruth saw Theo had also left the door open, a pet peeve, her jaw clenched, and she. . . .

In that precious moment Ruth has a choice: *a choice moment.* Ruth can gently close the door, welcome Theo, and make a note to check in with him later. Or, she could slam the door and chew him out, as is her tendency. What does Ruth do? What would you do? And does Ruth really have a choice, or is she caught in "knee-jerk mode"?

Responding in healthy ways to stressful situations—*response-ability*—is a vital aspect of resilience and well-being. Response-ability starts with recognizing our automatic reactions, and ultimately includes the ability to *choose responses* in choice moments (like gently closing the door). Responses rock: they tend to produce heightened wellness and resilience. Reactions typically suck: they mostly make things worse and reinforce the reaction itself. Ruth's door-slamming reaction precludes her from learning what is going on with Theo, adds stress to the classroom, and just reinforces her angry habit.

Freezing, fighting, fleeing, fawning, and fainting (see table 5.2) are common reactions rooted in survival instincts. Any significant threat, or even a reminder of one, can trigger a reaction that the brain barely knows is happening. But these snap reactions are a natural and sometimes life-saving part of being human, so some gratitude and self-compassion are in order. Dodging a ball heading for your face is a great choice we're grateful the brain didn't have to make. Mouthing off at the vice principal is a not-so-great choice we would like our brain to save us from. Both reactions show we're human.

Nurture reinforces this nature through coping behavior learned in early life. For example, living with someone who clams up and walks away in provoking situations, or flies into a rage, imprints our own reactions one way or another. Implicit biases can also be programmed from media-perpetuated stereotypes or prejudice that runs in a family. A black student arriving late might get treated differently from a white one. A female student may be steered away from science without conscious knowledge of the bias that influenced the behavior.

It takes time, awareness, and self-love to work with choice moments, as many reactions are literally tied to survival, and come with emotional flooding that shuts down thinking. However, with practice and kindness to self, students and teachers can develop response-ability through two miraculous stages, explored in this activity and the next:

1. Becoming aware of stressful moments ("choice moments") and our typical reactions.
2. Practicing regulation and choosing healthy responses in the midst of a choice moment.

Working at either stage produces more awareness, self-compassion, and gratitude to fuel continued growth and development of response-ability.

Developing the first stage is the focus of this activity, which boosts the chance for the second stage to occur. Life's choice moments may be stressful, but they are also opportunities to practice response-ability, boosting resilience and wellness.

Summary: Notice and reflect on stressful events to become more aware of habitual reactions.
Time: 15 minutes (initial), 5 minutes × 3 (ongoing)
Trust Required: High

1. *Prep* (optional): Print copies of table 5.2 "Response-Ability" for students, or display it to the class. Consider using "Taking Refuge" (p. 17) throughout the discussion to help with self-regulation.
2. *Choice Moment* (5 minutes): Share an example when you as a teacher automatically reacted to a "choice moment," which was mild or moderate, not severe. For example, cursing in traffic or fleeing an intense discussion. Ask students if they can think of their own examples, keeping in mind that student sharing is always optional.
3. *Reacting* (5 minutes): Introduce table 5.2 to students making connections between the examples shared and the information in the first column (REACTING). For example, seeing

cursing as a fight response. Explore the different ways bodies, hearts, and minds respond to stress (freeze, fight, flight, and so on). Emphasize that none of these are inherently bad or shameful because they are:
   a. hardwired for survival purposes (so sometimes crucially important) and
   b. often learned "no-fault" through early influences and coping patterns.
4. *Recognizing Lifeplay* (5 minutes): Invite students to watch for their personal reactions to stress or perceived threats over the next week or two, committing as a teacher to doing the same. Table 5.2 can be used to keep notes and highlight *reactions* (such as going silent) or telltale signs in the *recognizing* column (such as increased heart rate). Teach students that awareness builds in a progression (refer to the bottom of table 5.2), although there may be many experiences of *regulating* and *responding* to discuss as well. There is no need to share anything at this point, although students may wish to do so.
5. *Debrief* (5 minutes × 3–4 times): Periodically invite sharing about the lifeplay to see what happened when students tried to notice and reflect on stressful incidents and reactions, and remind any who may have forgotten about the lifeplay.
   a. Draw out observations, thoughts, feelings, changes, or impacts.
   b. Refer to and discuss various elements of the response-ability chart (see table 5.2) to build familiarity and some comfort in stressful situations. Encourage a deeper exploration of response-ability by spending some time on the RECOGNIZING, REGULATING, and RESPONDING columns, not just REACTING.
   c. Invite self-reflection along a continuum of awareness (see bottom of table 5.2), being willing to share as a teacher first (students do not have to). Ask if anything has changed in terms of their awareness of stressful moments and reactions.

6. *Integration Strategy*: Classrooms provide many choice moments, for example, a fire drill, announcing a test, or getting a new class assigned as a teacher. Watch for, acknowledge, and talk about these moments as they arise, along with accompanying reactions or responses. Explore all the columns, but praise the awareness of any of them, for this is deep work. Doing this in the context of classroom life directly grows resilience traits and emotional well-being.
7. *Safety*: Avoid abuse, self-harm, or other traumatic events as examples. Instead, bring up mild to moderately stressful moments typically experienced by most people. Some students (e.g., with severe trauma) may need to take a break or walk, talk to a friend, or even skip the activity. In any case, discussing reaction modes could cause distress. It may help to give a content warning (see p. 52) and seek input from students (anonymously) prior to engaging in any activity that might reasonably be upsetting or triggering.

Keywords: caring, cognitive, emotional, empower, lifeplay, mindfulness, resilience, safety, support

Table 5.2. Response-Ability to Stressful Situations (Choice Moments)

	Reacting	Recognizing	Regulating	Responding
What is it?	Automatically acting in the midst of a threat, stress, or trigger, without thought.	Noticing stressful moments and our reactions: (a) after they occur; (b) while they occur; (c) before they occur.	Moderating intense emotions, or our responses to stressful moments, on purpose.	Choosing a healthy, wise, loving response to a stressful moment or threat.
Why do it?	Helps with survival but can also reduce wellness where reactions are too frequent, intense or inappropriate.	Gives perspective on situations *and* a chance to move to REGULATING or RESPONDING.	Reduces the intensity of emotional, mental or physical distress, increasing the chance for RESPONDING.	Gives options for healthier, more positive choices leading to wellness for self and others.

Table 5.2. *(continued)*

	Reacting	Recognizing	Regulating	Responding
How to get more of it?	We generally don't benefit from more reactions (which we are born with and are shaped by early influences or coping patterns).	Develop awareness AND knowledge of the REACTING column AND the symptoms below, especially the rows which are habitual.	Do everything in the box at left (←), AND celebrate and practice the skill of RECOGNIZING, especially the "while they occur" part.	Do everything in the box at left (←), AND celebrate and practice the skills in the REGULATING column AND have self-compassion.
Freeze	• shutting down involuntarily • numbing • not speaking • not acting • not moving • spacing out • not deciding	Being aware of: • fear, butterflies • hyper alertness • stiffness, numbness • tension in body • dry mouth • pit in stomach • heart rate changes • breath changes	Take slow, deep breaths. Move your head, limbs, or body. Sing a song, eat, or drink. Open a window. Rub the hands or face. Focus intently on your surroundings. Take a break/walk or find some safe support.	Sometimes, the heightened awareness of freeze helps us pause and assess, hide from real danger, or come to full awareness. Mostly, regulating freeze allows a wider choice of healthier responses.
Fight	• constantly ready to fight • aggressive, bullying behavior • blaming, controlling, demanding • attacking others, shouting • spreading lies or silent treatment • attacking self	Being aware of: • anger, aggression • urge to hit, kick, injure • loud voice • wide, glaring eyes • clenched jaw, fists • muscle tension • knotted guts • rapid, shallow breaths	Take slow, deep, breaths. Douse the face or dunk the head in water. Use an ice pack. Take 10 breaths, 10 minutes, or 24 hours. Exercise, take a break/walk or find some safe support.	Sometimes, fight may be healthy to get clarity on toxic situations, protect self and others assertively, or fight a real danger. Mostly, regulating fight allows a wider choice of healthier responses.

	Reacting	Recognizing	Regulating	Responding
Flight	• running away • avoiding a talk, place, problem or person • cannot be still, nervous moving • perfectionism • escape into work, loud music, etc.	Being aware of: • anxiety • sharpened hearing • faster heart rate and breathing • nervous, restless movements of eyes, body, feet • feeling trapped • desire to run • trembling	Take slow, deep, breaths. Plant the feet firmly or hold onto something. Take a break or find some safe support.	Sometimes, flight is healthy to leave toxic relationships and situations, or flee a real danger. Mostly, regulating flight allows a wider choice of healthier responses.
Fawn	• pleasing, flattery, appeasing • can't say no • codependence • excessive apologizing and taking blame • forfeiting needs, rights, desires, or boundaries	Being aware of: • anxiety, guilt • eyes averted, head bowed • smiling, nodding • saying yes, agreeing • feeling responsible • not knowing one's own feelings	Take slow, deep, breaths. Tune into the deepest values in the heart. Practice being with the upset of others. Recognize core feelings, desires, boundaries, and speak them. Take a break or find some safe support.	Sometimes, it may be healthy to fawn by distracting with a compliment, come to a fair compromise, or have empathy. Mostly, regulating fawn allows a wider choice of healthier responses.
Faint, Flop, Flag	• collapsing, even when not tired • quitting quickly or automatically when things get challenging • fainting • dissociating	Being aware of: • feeling overly down or bored • head lowering • eyes closing • lightness in the head	Take deep breaths. Move your head, limbs or body. Rub the hands or face. Take a break or find some safe support.	Sometimes, it may be healthy to disengage when a break is needed, give up on a hopeless situation, or go limp with a threat. Mostly, regulating faint, flop or flag allows a wider choice of healthier responses.

Table 5.2. (continued)

	Reacting	Recognizing	Regulating	Responding
Notes				

Continuum of Awareness and Response-Ability

Awareness of Stressful Moments & Reactions	Response-Ability
No awareness of the moment or reaction.	No response (reaction only).
Awareness comes hours or days after.	Think of a response hours or days after.
Awareness comes minutes or seconds after.	Think of a response minutes or seconds after.
Awareness during the moment/reaction.	Change reaction to a response mid-moment.
Deep awareness during the moment/reaction.	Choose a response mid-moment.
Anticipate reactions before they happen.	Plan a response ahead of an anticipated moment.

Response-Ability Part 2: Using Life to Free Yourself (Main Move)

> "Surrender is the most difficult thing in the world while you are doing it and the easiest when it is done."
>
> —Bhai Sahib

We've all had the experience of something setting us off. Stored pain from the past can be activated by a sight, sound, or thought today. Being activated in this way can be overwhelming, resulting in reactions that are out of proportion to otherwise manageable life situations. The key is practicing loving responses to stressful situations, such as a big test in a difficult school subject.

Some may try to avoid such discomfort before it happens, for example by not signing up for said scary subject. While moving away from bad things can be healthy (even amoebas do it), such choices might limit life opportunities. Avoiding, distracting, numbing, or repressing short-term leads to long-term unwellness. Instead, life's challenges can become opportunities to make loving responses (see "RESPONDING" in table 5.2) and cultivate long-term freedom. Some example responses, in the context of the test scenario, could be

- regulating anxiety (see "REGULATING" in table 5.2) by taking a few long breaths;
- focusing on a more positive or helpful aspect: *"I've done well before; I can study"*;
- taking healthy action, like putting the test date and four study dates in a calendar (p. 171);
- self-soothing with music, happy photos, and stuffed animals while studying;
- taking refuge (p. 17) or practicing a mindful moment (p. 145) during the test;
- initiating self-care (p. 220) by taking a break when tired; and/or
- getting support from family, friends, or asking the teacher for some extra help.

However we respond, just accepting difficult emotions is a key trait of resilience (see table 5.1). When we feel stable and supported by such habits in easier times, we can come alongside ourselves lovingly in harder times. Cultivating self-kindness, presence, and self-compassion can release pain and increase well-being. Any time spent on this activity will be more than made up for in the reclamation of time lost to reactions and dealing with the fallout of destructive reactions. Young students can especially benefit, as they mature in an emotional phase of life.

Whether the critical stage of *recognizing* has been explored in "Response-Ability Part 1" or not, this "Part 2" cultivates both *recognizing* and a second miraculous stage of "response-ability": *responding* (instead of knee-jerking). Linda Graham describes response-ability as "response flexibility . . . the ability to pause, step back, reflect, shift perspectives, create options and choose wisely."[10] This activity provides acronyms (handout 5.3) that grow resilience traits (see table 5.1) while transforming the everyday stress of life, and classroom life, into wellness.

> **Summary**: Use acronyms as reminders to transform challenging experiences into wellness.
> **Time**: 15 minutes (initial), 5 minutes (repeated debriefs).
> **Trust Required**: High
>
> 1. *Prep*: As a teacher, choose one of the acronyms from handout 5.3 and use it in your own life for a few weeks or more. Use the acronym as many times as you can remember in school, at home, and elsewhere. Proceed to step 2 once you have developed some personal familiarity with using the acronym to work with difficult emotions/experiences.
> 2. *Share* (5 minutes): Share with students a personal experience of feeling *mildly* stressed or challenged (e.g., meeting a deadline). Invite them to do the same, perhaps in a circle (see p. 57), but always with the freedom to respond or not. Share as much contextual information from the introduction above as you feel is appropriate for your class. Allow time for any comments and discussion.

3. *Demonstrate* (2 minutes): Walk students through the acronym you used in steps 1 and 2, describing how it works for you, how you have changed from using it, and any other personal aspect that resonates. Teacher credibility and lived experience is powerful.
4. *Choose Acronym* (5 minutes): Share handout 5.3 with students. Have them find an acronym that resonates for them, and write it down or keep it somewhere prominent.
5. *Lifeplay* (3 minutes): Invite students to use the acronym whenever life challenges them. Highlight the importance of remembering: becoming aware enough to actually disrupt a stress reaction is the heart of the practice.
6. *Debriefs* (5 minutes × 5+): Each day for a week, and then weekly afterward, remind the class about the acronym and solicit a few stories, transformations, or insights, including yours as a teacher. Revisit table 5.2 and the continuum at the bottom to note changes.
7. *Integration Strategy*: Use the acronym in any classroom. Teachers and young people can have surprisingly similar stress: new material, a big presentation, getting bumped in the hallway, deadlines, and (of course) the student at the front who breathes too loud.
8. *Safety*: Intense triggers are a harmful aftereffect of trauma. While this activity has the potential to transform less serious triggers into T.R.I.G.G.E.R.S. (timely, rewarding, invaluable gifts granting eternal release and salvation), it is intended for use with everyday stress. Introduce this activity in the context of *mild* challenges in life. In time, you may feel comfortable encouraging students to use their acronym for more difficult experiences (some may do this regardless). Consider checking in with school or district support staff to enlist their support with the activity.

Keywords: card, caring, choice, cognitive, circle, emotional, empower, foundational, integration, lifeplay, mindfulness, resilience, safety, spiritual, time-maker

Handout 5.3. Using Life to Free Yourself
Name: _____

1) Read the acronyms below to find one that resonates with you, or make up your own.
2) Write it on a slip of paper, flower petal, your hand: anywhere prominent to remind you.
3) When life challenges you, try to remember to use the acronym steps. This is everything.
4) With practice—dozens or hundreds of times—notice what changes as life frees you.

A	*Awareness* and *acknowledgement* that something difficult is happening.
D	*Deep breath* and *deepen* into your body feelings with a soft, kind-hearted awareness.
A	*Accept* whatever you find inside, as well as your capability to accept, or not.
P	*Praise* yourself to celebrate the noticing of something difficult and adapting to it.
T	*Thrive* in a healthy response, knowing you are developing your capacity to adapt.

P	*Pause* everything.
R	*Relax* your body.
O	*Open* your heart.
G	*Green-light* whatever is happening.
R	*Release* anything that wants letting go.
E	*Embrace* yourself kindly, holding wherever you need it most.
S	*Select* a healthy response to the situation, if appropriate.
S	*Smile* in celebration of the progress you are making or *share* with a friend.

R	*Remember* you have a choice.
E	*Enlarge* your heart and awareness around what's happening.
D	*Dream* or *Do* a wise, skillful, loving response.
O	*Open* your heart to let go of outcomes OR *Offer* your response without expectation.

R	*Recognize* your stressed state (and notice how recognition alone softens things).
E	*Exhale* deeply (and your exhale will require a deep inhale as well).
S	*Sense* the feelings and your body (without putting any energy into thinking).
E	*Express* gratitude to yourself and the moment (for transforming stress into grace).
T	*Take* wise, loving action, if needed (bringing wisdom and wellness to the situation).

S	*Stop/sense/silence* . . . breathe, feel your body and listen with love.
H	*Honor* whatever you notice is there, welcoming it as a passing guest.
I	*Inquire* as to what might serve your highest need or well-being at this time.
F	*Find* a way to give what you need to yourself (if not now, at some time).
T	*Thank* yourself, others, and the experience . . . for the gift of shift.

Here are some popular response-ability acronyms; does one resonate for you?

- STOP—Stop, Take Breaths, Observe, Proceed[11]
- RAIN—Recognition, Accept/Acknowledge/Allow, Interest, Non-Identification[12]
- RAIN—Recognize, Allow, Investigate, Nurture[13]
- PAUSE—Paying Attention Unveils Sacred Experiences[14]
- RRR—Recognize (self-awareness), Respond (self-expression), Reset (self-care)[15]
- SBNRR (SiBerian North RailRoad)—Stop, Breathe, Notice, Reflect, Respond[16]

Could Be Good, Could Be Bad

"Where one door is shut, another is opened."[17]

—Miguel de Cervantes

A proverb tells of a farmer who lost a runaway horse. When a neighbor came by to offer sympathy for the loss, the farmer said, "Could be good, could be bad." The next day, the horse returned with seven other wild horses. The neighbor was happy for the farmer's good fortune, but the farmer again only said, "Could be good, could be bad." A day later, the farmer's son broke his leg trying to tame one of the horses. The neighbor offered condolences, to which the farmer replied, "Could be good, could be bad." The day after that, the army came to conscript young people for the war, but they left the farmer's son at home due to his injury.

Life is a mystery, both in the grief of losing the beloved and meaningful but also in how loss opens doors to growth and wellness. This wellness isn't in the form of joy, but in the destinations found on the pathways of crisis: more life appreciation, better relationships, shifted priorities, appreciation of personal strengths, and a richer spiritual life.[18] This activity helps students and teachers appreciate the good that comes with the bad, the bad with the good, and gain a little more resilience in smoothing out life's ups and downs.

Summary: Soften perspectives on what is perceived as good or bad.
Time: 12 minutes
Trust Required: Medium

1. *Introduction* (1 minute): Tell the farmer story, or briefly explore the meaning of the yin yang symbol (☯) as opposites being contained within each other.
2. *T-Chart* (3 minutes): Invite students to write a few examples of "good" and "bad" things from their own lives on a T-chart. The list is private, and the teacher, as always, completes their own list. Use "mildly good" or "mildly bad" for a safer activity.
3. *Yin Yang* (4 minutes): Now challenge students to write down something good (e.g., some new learning, growth, or an opportunity) that relates to, or might have come out of, each "bad" thing on the list. For example, botching a test may lead to better study habits. Parents divorcing may bring a peaceful home. Invite the class to do the same with the "good" list, writing down something not so good associated with each item. For example, getting an A+ once but then feeling anxious because high grades became a parental expectation.
4. *Debrief* (5 minutes): Use the standard debrief questions (p. 16), and then prompt with the following:
   a. How was it for you to look for the good in the bad, or the bad in the good?
   b. Is seeing the good in the bad the same thing as minimizing a loss?
   c. What is gained from one door closing? What can we learn from failure? What are the opportunities inherent in challenge and adversity?
5. *Safety*: Students experiencing a recent, significant loss may be upset and/or unable to find redeeming factors early in the process. Acknowledge this, and allow the use of non-personal examples or focus only on milder events.
6. *Integration Strategy*: Run this activity in the aftermath of a particularly challenging lesson, test, unit, or any (non-traumatic) setback in a class. Look for curriculum connec-

> tions wherever there is evaluation, critical thinking, or judgment in good or bad.
> **Keywords**: caring, emotional, gratitude, integration, prep-free, resilience, spiritual, support

Help Wanted Microlab

"Support yourself and heaven will help you."

—Senegalese Proverb

Two trains leave the station, one travels east at 80 km/h, one travels west at . . . sound familiar? Sound engaging? How many not-so-relevant problems do students get like this?[19] How many problems do they work with in class that are pertinent to their personal, real lives? This activity invites students to explore real-world problems with a focus on the core skills of resilience.

This exploration is aided with a hidden treasure trove of wisdom and resourcefulness that can help with virtually any problem imaginable: the students in the room. Whatever challenge might be posed, big or small, this incredible store of resilience and good sense is ready, waiting, and available. Teachers pose a challenge and facilitate the student sharing using a microlab to practice and explore the traits of resilience.

> **Summary**: Students respond to anonymous challenges in a microlab format.
> **Time**: 25 minutes
> **Trust Required**: Medium
>
> 1. *Prep* (5 minutes): Choose a topic to work with using any or all of these methods:
>   a. pick one of "not succeeding in school" or "not or making a school team";
>   b. seek anonymous suggestions (p. 40) from students such as "a friend snubs you";
>   c. ask a vice principal, school counselor, or social worker for an appropriate topic; or

d. write a problem statement based on one of the following topics: "I worry that my parents can't afford to pay for school after high school" or "I spend too much time scrolling on my phone and feel bad afterward."
- academic pressure
- alcohol, smoking, drugs
- anxiety
- body image
- bullying/cyberbullying
- climate crisis
- coping with stress
- depression
- diet/sleep
- discrimination
- emotional changes
- family conflict
- financial security
- mental health
- obesity
- pandemic
- personal safety
- physical changes/health
- poverty
- social issues
- risk-taking
- school/study problems
- self-esteem
- separation/divorce
- sexual health
- technology addiction
- violence/war

2. *Microlab* (15–20 minutes): Put students in groups of 3, lettering off A, B, and C, and give them table 5.1 as a reference. Display the chosen problem to the class and explain that students will respond to it using the traits of resilience. They can pretend they are guiding a good friend who has this problem, hence the name "help wanted microlab." Explain the following microlab rotation, and use a timer to prompt students through these steps:
   a. quiet thinking time for everyone in the room to reflect on the problem and the traits of resilience to find connections (2 minutes);
   b. person A in each group shares, while B and C listen mindfully (1–2 minutes);
   c. silent reflection (15–30 seconds);
   d. person B in each group shares, while A and C listen mindfully (1–2 minutes);
   e. silent reflection (15–30 seconds);
   f. person C in each group shares, while A and B listen mindfully (1–2 minutes);
   g. silent reflection (15–30 seconds);

h. free discussion within small groups, ending with thanks to partners (2 minutes); and
   i. debrief as a whole class, drawing out ideas heard in the groups, and any feelings, impact, or connections made.
3. *Safety*: Students may identify with a problem, however it is chosen, and feel a corresponding intensity. As with any activity, students can take refuge (p. 17) when needed, or use other strategies listed in the safety section there (p. 21).
4. *Integration Strategy*: Microlab can be applied to any curricular challenge, thorny discussion topic, or problem, reducing the trust required to "low." Incorporate the traits of resilience as a reference in your curriculum work. For example, in exploring how communities have adapted to their geographic environment or how drama students improvise for a scene. School-based challenges also require less trust, such as how to display school awards in the halls or address climate change through a local school program.
5. *Lifeplay*: If the microlab is repeated, students may feel safe enough to begin suggesting life problems anonymously, which the whole class can then microlab—powerful stuff.

Keywords: caring, collaborative, choice, empower, lifeplay, resilience, support

Lifeline Graphs

"You may not control all the events that happen to you, but you can decide not to be reduced by them."[20]

—Maya Angelou

Life's challenges are often hidden beneath a smiling exterior, with social media creating a major gap between reality and retweets. Scrolling through the "perfect" online lives of others can leave students feeling like they are the only ones with problems. Confronting this myth in sensitive ways (see the story of the teacher circle on p. 112) can normalize the sharing of challenges, along with our healthy responses to them—both key traits for resilience.

Summary: Students sketch a line representing life's ups and downs, and discuss.
Time: 10 minutes
Trust Required: Varies

1. *Draw* (2 minutes): Invite students to draw a line representing the ups and downs of their life (medium trust) or a famous person (low trust). Time is on the horizontal axis with life highs and lows shown in the vertical dimension. *Assure students that there will be no requirement to show their lifeline or talk about it unless they wish to.* Students can choose to represent their entire lives or choose a particular period. Lifelines often look something like a roller coaster. Teachers may sketch their own example on a whiteboard or screen while narrating some aspect of their own life, or they may choose not to give students any influence around what a lifeline "should" look like.
2. *Personal Reflection* (1 minute): When students have finished drawing their line, give them a minute to reflect on highs, lows, or anything that stands out on the line.
3. *Partner Share* (2 minutes, optional): Have students share their lifeline with a partner.
4. *Reveal* (1 minute, optional): Invite students to reveal their lifeline at the same time, if they wish. Give a 3-2-1 countdown and those who wish to may hold up their lifeline.
5. *Debrief* (6 minutes): The following prompts may be helpful in debriefing the activity:
   a. What strikes you about people's lifelines?
   b. What were your thoughts and feelings as you drew your lifeline?
   c. Would anyone like to share about where their line went up or changed from a down? What contributed to the change?
   d. What are the drawbacks of the "ups" or the benefits of the "downs"?
   e. Can a line be only "up"? What does "up" mean if there is no "down"?

6. *Integration Strategy*: Lines and functions are core aspects of grade 7–12 mathematics and have many potential connections: axis labels, positive or negative slopes, rates of change, maximum and minimum points, and tangents all have meaning in both math and life. Students can be given the option to create a timeline for a famous person from any course (art, history, civics, and more) with a resilience story (e.g., Martin Luther King Jr.).
7. *Safety*: Students can self-adjust for safety by sketching the life of a famous person (instead of their own), or writing instead of drawing. Sharing is always optional, and since students may feel awkward if they are the only ones not sharing, poll the class anonymously (p. 40) to see how many want to share. This activity requires a minimum of medium trust as a baseline and high trust for the sharing of personal lifelines.

Keywords: card, caring, creative, emotional, eudaimonia, growth, integration, prep-free, resilience, short-'n'-safe

Repairing (Almost) Anything: Restoration for Resilience

"The circle is a way in which community is made and remade . . . each person is considered the beginning and end of the circle and holds the task of asking for the highest truth for the wellbeing of the community."

—Orland Bishop

The most skillful conflict resolution strategy ever is to avoid conflict in the first place. Two such proactive approaches, relationship building (see p. 55) and emotional regulation (p. 184), boost wellness and head off interpersonal strife. Inevitably however, conflict *will* arise. From a hurtful comment in the foyer to a fight about group workload, this activity reworks "Table 1.1: Questions to Debrief Anything" to "Table 5.4: Questions to Repair (Almost) Anything."

Since interpersonal (and intrapersonal) fractures lie at the core of most issues, the healing of relationships is at the heart of restoration. For this reason, those who have caused the harm as well as those impacted by it, and sometimes others from the community, participate in the question dialogue.[21] Dictating punishment from a place of authority does little to prevent future problems, but engaging everyone involved builds lifelong skills to repair harm from conflict.

Formal restorative circles are conducted by trained restorative practices (RP) facilitators.[22] Yet regular teachers and students can use table 5.4 to guide the exploration of conflicts, repair harm, restore relationship harmony in the classroom, and teach vital resilience skills to students.

As teachers will also follow their local school or district behavior codes, this process can complement such protocols. Repairing harm requires all stakeholders to personally engage, become accountable for what happened, and co-construct what could change to make things better. When used in conjunction with a circle, the result is literally a relationship-strengthening cycle that can foster peace and wellness in any group.

Table 5.4. Questions to Repair (Almost) Anything

During Incident	After Incident	Intended Responses
What is happening?	What happened?	Sensory impressions of the incident: what was seen or heard without other commentary.
What are you thinking?	What were you thinking?	Thoughts about the incident: delving into the cognitive domain.
What are you feeling?	What were you feeling?	Feelings about the incident: delving into the emotional domain.
What is the impact?	What was the impact?	Impacts of the experience on self, perceived impacts on others, groups, situations, property, the environment, etc.
Is there any meaning, growth, or connection to find in this?		Mining the incident for eudaimonic aspects of meaning and growth, as well as connections to school or life.
What *could* change in a good way?		Ideas to show remorse, change personal behavior, make restitution, or anything else that might bring deeper wellness to the situation, others, and self.

Summary: Use questions to repair (almost) any classroom or school conflict.
Time: Varies
Trust Required: Varies

1. *Prep* (2 minutes): Copy the questions (table 5.4) for students and teachers to carry around. Spend some time as a teacher using the questions in a variety of contexts below, ranging from less involved to more involved situations. Eventually, students will use the questions with each other in these contexts as well.
2. *"I" Statements* (low trust required) can be used by any member of the school community:
   a. Start with "I" and what happened: "I hear you interrupting Alexa . . .
   b. Followed with a thought or feeling: "and I wonder if you respect her . . .
   c. Then the impact: "because everyone needs to feel like they will be heard."
   d. Then ask for a change that would help: "I need you to listen when others speak."
   e. And an invitation to talk: "Can you talk to me about this?"
   f. Use table 5.4 to continue the dialogue until a way forward is agreed on, such as "I'm sorry, I won't interrupt; and I'll ask for the talking piece in future."
3. *Restorative Talks* (medium trust required) are informal one-on-one or small group dialogues where the questions are used in the context of an incident (such as a hallway imsult). Gather everyone involved in a small circle and work the questions from top to bottom. The parties involved can ask each other the questions or a third party (usually a teacher) can facilitate. Sometimes it helps to linger on a particular question to dig deeper into that aspect. For example, ask repeatedly about impact to get nuances of impact on those involved, those not present, long-term impacts, and more.

4. *Peace Paths* (medium trust required) involve posting the questions along a wall at eye level or on the floor of the classroom. This provides a restorative space where two people can go to resolve a conflict by walking the path of the questions together, one by one. *Search terms*: peace path.
5. *Restorative Circles* (high trust required) use a community circle to involve more stakeholders, including those involved in the incident, supporters of those involved, or others in the school community. These larger circles can resolve whole-class incidents or more complex conflicts. Formal circle agreements and a talking piece help, as does having students bring their questions to the circle for reference. The teacher will facilitate, moving from person to person through each question in a flexible manner that ensures all voices are heard. Come back to the questions over and over. A vital outcome is reaching consensus agreement about the final question: what change needs to happen in a good way? Some examples follow:
    a. A whole class circle to discuss students constantly packing up early and waiting around for the bell, or the teacher taking a long time to return student assignments (yes, teachers need to be held accountable and share power in this process).
    b. A circle of students involving a bully, the bullied, a bystander, supporters for the bullied, and potentially a teacher supporter for the bully as well. School administration can also be involved in such circles.
    c. A student who plagiarized work in dialogue with the teacher, someone close to and supportive of the student, and another teacher of the same subject or grade.
6. *Lifeplay* (5 minutes): Invite students to carry the questions with them and use them any time they are involved in a dispute or disagreement: at home, in clubs or teams, or anywhere. Encourage this as a teacher by using the questions often and publicly, helping strengthen resilience in the entire classroom community.

7. *Debrief* (5 minutes): Periodically ask students whether and how they are using the questions using the standard debrief questions (table 1.1).
8. *Safety*: Teachers must remain ultimately responsible for classroom behavior and school discipline protocols. Ensure students have some confidence and practice with the questions before inviting them to use them on their own, or facilitate restorative situations in class, perhaps using a fishbowl (p. 190), to build the practice.
9. *Schoolwide Extension / Integration Strategy*: Where traditional punitive measures such as detentions or suspensions are a part of most schools' disciplinary frameworks, a restorative approach may become a complement, and training can be sought.[23] Once a teacher has developed a deep comfort repairing harm, they may help other staff repair harm with their students, creating a schoolwide approach to conflict that builds skills of resilience and well-being together.

Keywords: circle, collaborative, emotional, empower, integration, lifeplay, resilience, restorative, safety, schoolwide

SUPPLEMENTARIES: SHORT, SIMPLE, SAFE, OR SEARCHABLE RESILIENCE

- *Ask Three, Then Me* encourages students to ask three peers for help first before seeking out the teacher, building a wider network of support for academic and other needs.
- *Character Traits (Integrated Strategy)* invites students to use table 5.1 to identify and discuss various traits of resilience found in characters they encounter in the fiction or nonfiction they read in school.
- *Circles of Resilience* invites students to map their life situations within circles of *control, influence,* or *acceptance.* Discuss figure 5.1 with students after inviting them to put some examples from

their life on it to help them develop a key trait of resilience. *If you have control of something, no worries. If you don't . . . no worries.*
- Does everything in your life fit on here in one way or another?
- Where do your challenges fall in these circles?
- Is there anything you actually have *complete* control over?
- In which circle(s) do the things you think about go?
- In which circle(s) do you spend time and effort doing things?

• *"Giving. Up"* dispels the socially conditioned myth to "never give up." In some intractable situations, when everything in one's power has been tried to no avail, continued effort, energy, or time spent may be pointless, unhealthy, or even self-destructive. *Giving* means to free oneself. *Up* means to move onward and upward to something else. Help students see that letting go of a particular outcome can be a wise, self-loving gift rather than be seen as a failure.

• *Opening Hope* involves the exploration and cultivation of hope: a key trait for resilience. Students can discuss the following prompts in circle or as part of a writing or art task:
- Can you list (or draw) some things you hope for?

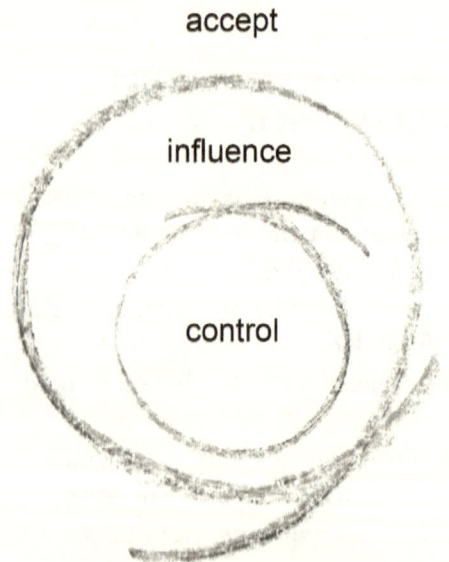

Figure 5.1. Circles of Resilience

- Was there a time when you had (or didn't have) hope? What happened?
- Where can hope come from?
- If our sense of hope can change, how could you get more in your life?
- *Inner Caring Committee* is a mental process from Rick Hanson to imagine an inner support team of three to five people, characters, animals, or any beings (alive or not, real or not).[24] These team members will evoke the qualities most desired by the student: safety, supportiveness, strength, resilience, compassion, caring, wisdom, and so on. This team can be summoned in times of need. *Search terms*: caring, committee.
- *Mindfulness* activities (see p. 145) listed in the cognitive domain all contribute to resilience through the development of acceptance and equanimity in the face of challenges.
- *Resilientences* turn self-defeating phrases into more resilient ones. Also see Watched Word (p. 173) for another take on this. Here are some examples of "resilientences":
  - "Yet" can be added to a sentence as in "I don't understand, *yet*." or "I can't do that . . . yet." Carol Dweck introduced the power of "yet," to reframe challenges.[25]
  - "And" can be used instead of "but" to soften resistance and add a willingness to build onto challenging ideas rather than oppose them. For example, "Yes, the due date is tomorrow, *and* reworking this section seems critical."
  - "I am getting better at this" replaces "I suck at this" or "I'll never get it."
  - "I'll try again," "I can break this into steps," "It may take time," "I'll get help," or "What am I missing?" can replace self-defeating words like "I can't," "It's too hard," "I'm stupid," and so forth.
  - Teachers can also avoid the words "yes" and "no" in responding to student questions in order for students to develop their own capacity to trust and verify what is right and wrong for themselves. For example, in reply to "Ms. Duarte, is the area 54 cm^2?" say "Why do you think it's 54?" or "How could it be 54?"
- *Self-Talk Team Turnaround* invites seven classroom volunteers to stand in a line at the front of class to role-play positive and

negative self-talk. Give the student in the middle a card with a starting thought. They then read it as though having the thought themselves:
- "Hmm, I've got a big test tomorrow!"
- "Hmm, I like this shirt, but should I wear it today?"
- "Hmm, soccer tryouts start next week."
- "Hmm, look at that zit!"
- [Insert your own youth situation here].

The three students on their left then think up, and speak aloud, negative self-talk responses. Those on the right give positive options that a loving, caring friend or coach might say. When the six are done, ask for other examples from the class, then the student in the middle gets the last word. Discuss the impact of negative self-talk: mental comparisons, self-judgments, and/or self-criticisms. Then explore how positive turnarounds can lead to self-compassion and self-love. Students may have difficulty thinking of positive self-talk, so give examples (recognizing negativity bias, finding small areas of improvement, accepting imperfections as aspects of beauty, uniqueness, or vulnerability).

- *Stress Signals* has students in small groups tracing a body outline onto mural paper, and then drawing physical stress signals on the figure: sweaty palms, tingly solar plexus, hunched shoulders, tight jaw, and so on. Recognizing these signals is the first step in being able to have the option to choose an effective response (see Response-ability, p. 115) for much more.
- *Traits of Resilience* is a class discussion that can be held during or after an adverse (but not immediately traumatic) experience, whether it happened in or out of the classroom. Share table 5.1 with students and invite observations about which traits are most relevant for the particular experience and what students can do to practice them.
- *Three What's* asks students (and teacher) to reflect individually, in small groups, and/or as a whole class circle on three questions that explore personal life balance:

- What's something you could put more effort into?
- What's something you could be more patient with?
- What's something you could let go of completely?
- *Unstuck Posters* help students help themselves when they encounter a roadblock in the classroom by providing general solutions to try. *Search terms*: stuck, unstuck, classroom, poster, [image search].

6

COGNITIVE WELL-BEING

Mental and Intellectual Health

> "The one continuing purpose of education, since ancient times, has been to bring people to as full a realization as possible of what it is to be a human being. Other statements of educational purpose have also been widely accepted. . . . The broader humanistic purpose includes all of them, and goes beyond them, for it seeks to encompass all the dimensions of human experience."[1]
>
> —Arthur W. Foshay

Students all over the world (and many of their teachers) have questioned the purpose of school, mostly on stifling June afternoons. If they were given district mission statements to read, they would find the same top priority parroted most everywhere: academic achievement.[2] Citizenship typically comes next, along with whatever other ideals can be packed into a sentence. But for all these lofty goals, the bulk of what actually happens in schools is the stuffing of student minds with academic knowledge and skills.[3]

Policy makers contribute to the feeding frenzy with aggressive agendas to raise standards, including high-stakes, standardized assessments that often come with bar-raising legislation.[4] These policies and tests mostly fail to raise anything, except stress. During the "Reach for the Top" performance-raising initiative in the United States from 2009 to

2015, PISA scores in reading, math, and science all *decreased*.[5] Innovations such as twenty-first-century skills sound good, shifting efforts away from fact recall and skill grinding to critical thinking, creativity, and higher-order thinking. But these just represent different heights on a cognitive heap. This is not cognitive wellness but cognitive overload.

Mental health isn't just mental, despite the name, and despite the bias for thinking in education. This bias begins early, with students in most districts taking IQ tests at a young age that shape their school programs forever. Those programs include years of mandated learning in subjects chock full of cognitive knowledge or skills, with little or no legislated development in mental health or any other wellness domain. True cognitive wellness gives students ways to cope with these demands, while cultivating positive mental qualities like awareness and equanimity.

Hours after school ended, Paul was in a state of wonder about what happened in his grade 8 class that day. His teacher had been giving the class some mindfulness she had found online. Today's activity was to close the eyes and imagine a mouse hole with thoughts as mice. Paul had never been asked to think about his thinking, and when he tried this activity, there were some thoughts at first. But when he was told to watch the hole intently in his mind, an incredible moment came where there were no thoughts at all. What shocked Paul to the core was how good it felt, and how he could actually relax and not have a thought from time to time.

Student thriving will require a sea change in schools, moving from cognitive cramming to cognitive wellness (with a balanced diet of other well-being domains). The cognitive domain is one of many colors in the well-being palette and includes not just the head brain but the heart brain and gut brain as well.[6] If education is going to paint a picture of flourishing, it must use more than one color, or *any* color for that matter.

There is much that can be done at the school and classroom level to enact this cognitive transformation. The way we think links to our social, emotional, and physical well-being. It's vital to spend time exploring all these domains. In addition, to honor the deep interdependence of mind, body, and heart requires a shift from cognitive demand to cognitive well-being:

- nurturing and rewiring the all-precious brain, home of our mental life;

- exploring cognitive engagement and *flow*, finding optimally immersive states;[7] and
- developing metacognitive awareness and equanimity, key complements to cognition.

While cognitive well-being definitely increases academic achievement, its purpose isn't just to enable more learning. Learning how awareness works, building up practices of mental self-care, and understanding the cognitive states that lead to lasting fulfillment all contribute to well-being in multiple domains for those in or out of school.

Key Messages

- The ultimate aim of education is total human development, yet the primary focus in most schools is cognitive development, not cognitive wellness.
- A full-spectrum approach to well-being domains complements academic learning and overall wellness, including cognitive well-being.
- Metacognitive capacities of awareness, equanimity, self-directed neuroplasticity, and immersive cognitive states can be explicitly cultivated in the classroom.

COGNITIVE WELL-BEING ACTIVITIES

Mindfulness Moments Medley (Main Move)

"Everyday we are engaged in a miracle which we don't even recognise: a blue sky, white clouds, green leaves, the black, curious eyes of a child—our own two eyes. All is a miracle. Mindfulness is like that— it is the miracle which can call back in a flash our dispersed mind and restore it to wholeness so that we can live each minute of life."[8]

—Thích Nhất Hạnh

Learning places immense cognitive demands on students, with reams of curriculum, fact and skill memorization, problem-solving, and higher-order thinking. Students also expected to pay attention in countless ways, without ever being shown how. Similarly, they are expected to work collaboratively and deal with challenges, but are rarely taught the skills to do so. Mindfulness can help address these concerns, alleviating cognitive over-stuffing and helping students explore their own awareness and relationships to self and others.

Mindfulness is awareness, with acceptance, of senses, thoughts, and feelings in the present moment. Whether the awareness is directed inward, outward, or broadly diffused, it involves opening to whatever is experienced with acceptance. These aspects offer a host of well-being benefits for adolescents in multiple domains of well-being:[9]

- increased attention and reduced depression or anxiety (cognitive well-being);
- improved classroom climate and prosocial behavior (social well-being);
- better emotional regulation (emotional well-being);
- calmer responses to adversity and stress (resilience); and
- seeing a bigger picture beyond oneself (eudaimonic well-being).

Teachers also have much to gain if they participate in mindfulness as well as facilitate. This participation could involve formal practices like sitting meditation but also integrating mindful moments in movement, sensing the world, and daily classroom life. What's important, and powerful, is when teachers explore a practice themselves deeply and share that depth with others. While mindfulness can be many things, it is important to understand that it is *not*:

- a religion, though it has roots in many traditions;
- about suppressing thoughts or emotions, but accepting them with less judgment;
- mere passiveness, but engaging in life's decisions and actions with clarity;
- just paying attention, just being kind, or just relaxing, but a blend of these and more;
- only focusing on the good, but softening labeling of "good" and "bad" and
- breath meditation alone, but includes many other foci for those who need (see safety).

COGNITIVE WELL-BEING

This breadth of practice is reflected in the widespread adoption of mindfulness in the general population. The number of U.S. children meditating more than quadrupled from 2012 to 2017 and was evenly distributed by gender, race, and economic status. In fact, students in poorer families were actually more likely to use mindfulness.[10]

Though some students have experience with mindfulness, teachers may not feel confident leading it, or they may wonder about engagement. Third-party mindfulness programs, websites, and apps (often free for education) can help, providing lesson plans, guided practices, and more. This activity offers a smorgasbord of engaging, brief, and simple practices for developing mindful states, grouped by object of foci. Like Mindful Listening (p. 70) and Taking Refuge (p. 17), shorter mindful moments are readily integrated into daily life. Teachers can offer standard meditation, but brief techniques provide similar cognitive well-being benefits.[11]

Rotate these mindful moments each week on a wellness day or use them daily in class transitions. Try practicing solo as a teacher to bring personal insights when sharing with students.

Repetition with integrity and sincerity produces multiple shorter states that can contribute to long-term traits. For example, one deep breath may provide a moment of delicious calm, but repeated breaths carry that stability into more and more moments, cultivating a lasting spaciousness that permeates life, and balances the filling of minds with the stilling of minds.

> **Summary**: Explore an assortment of brief mindfulness moments or minutes with students.
> **Time**: 1–2 minutes (ongoing)
> **Trust Required**: Low
>
> 1. *Safety*: Some people feel more or less stable depending on the mindfulness focus chosen, due to body insecurities, trauma, or breathing issues. Use a variety of the focus categories below to help students find options that may feel more "at home" to them, and let them choose the best foci for them. See "Taking Refuge" safety (p. 21) for full details.

2. *Guidance*: Brief moments of mindfulness don't require much explanation, but these general points can help before, during, or after any of the practices.
    - Invite a curious, open stance to whatever happens: being rather than doing.
    - Stopping thoughts is not required as persistent thinking is typical. What helps is to not have any *intention* of thinking or add energy to thoughts that do pop up.
    - Rather than judging lapses during practice, encourage students to celebrate each return to awareness, as these are small victories on the road to cognitive wellness.
3. *Breath Moments* employ a most familiar mindfulness focus. Most of these practices use a natural flow of breath, so invite students to *receive* or *feel* the breath as it comes. This can help counteract the tendency to force the breath in some unnatural way.
    a. *Belly breaths* are taken with the hands covering the lower belly lovingly for three to five deep, calming cycles.
    b. *Counting breaths* is as simple as getting to ten, then starting again. If the count is lost, restart. Counting to three, or just "one, one, one, . . . may be more accessible.
    c. *Seven-eleven breathing* breathes in for a count of 7 seconds, and out for 11, which may have a relaxing effect. If the count feels long, students can try 5 and 9 seconds, or 3 and 5 durations, ultimately finding their own comfortable pace. Reversing the count (e.g., 11 inhales to 7 exhales) can have a stimulating and activating effect to awaken and sharpen senses.
    d. *One Deep Breath a Day* is a powerful practice that contains a challenge only a master can achieve: consistently *remembering* to take that one breath!
    e. *Drawing Breath (or Music)* uses pencil and paper to sketch an impression of the breath (or music) visually, while breathing (or listening). Finish after ten breaths, when the page is full, or until there is a feeling of completion.

f. *Square Breathing* draws four "sides" of a single breath cycle with the fingers in the air, or by imagining the square, whichever feels best. Count to four *inhaling* while drawing the left side of the square upward, then count four *holding* the breath to draw the top side, then to four *exhaling* for the right side, and the last four *holding* again to complete the bottom of the square, then repeat.

g. *Formal Breath Meditation* is to rest as awareness of the breath, keeping the breath company while allowing it to do whatever it wants, for longer periods of 5 minutes, 10 minutes, or longer. The guidance section in part 2 is vital for longer practice.

4. *Feel Moments* can be about external sensory touch or feeling the body itself, as mindfulness is not all in the head. Cultivating a gentle, accepting consciousness of the body cultivates the all-important physical and emotional dimensions of awareness.

a. *Just Feel* the world around you (air temperature, clothing, surfaces you are touching, etc.) and/or the world inside you (inner sensations/feelings in the body) without initiating thinking about what is felt and with a warm-hearted presence to whatever the body is sensing. Thoughts may come, but do not latch on to any such labeling, judging, or other mental commentary. Allow for the possibility of *becoming* feeling.

b. *Tracing Fingers* uses the thumb or finger of one hand to slowly trace the outline of the fingers on the other hand, moving *up* the finger on the inhale, *down* on the exhale. Swap to the other hand and repeat.

c. *Body Scans* don't have to be lengthy, although those are wonderful (see formal body meditation below). A brief head-to-toe scan can be quite refreshing, without any need to judge or mentally comment on what is found in the body.

d. *Soothing Touch* is any gesture done with feelings of self-love and the permission to relax. Each person can discover their own personal posture: a hand on the cheek, temple rub, face wash, neck massage, cross-armed self-hug, stretch, back of hand caress or folded hands. Over time, this private and personal touch can become a soothing and discreet practice of cognitive self-care.
e. *Inner Body Awareness* takes in the entire inner body all at once, letting go of thoughts, and merging deeply with the feeling or energy found inside. See *interoception* (p. 22) for more on this.
f. *Squeeze and Release* tenses one area of the body (e.g., hands, legs, face, back) firmly but slowly, then relaxes and releases that same part, all while staying aware of body sensations. Briefly work one area or progress through multiple parts, finishing with a whole-body squeeze and release, depending on what feels good.
g. *Finger Labyrinths* are freely available online for printing, and provide a tactile, soothing respite. Students may optionally write positive words (e.g., peace, acceptance, self-compassion, etc.) along the trail before they trace.
h. *Sole Focus* is to focus awareness on the soles of the feet as much as possible, for as long as feels comfortable, or until one feels grounded and relaxed.
i. *Mindful Sip/Bite* from a water bottle, mug, or any food (rather than a thoughtless gulp) cultivates the quality of awareness and absorption in sensing.
j. *Mystery Box* contains a variety of small objects such as feathers or trinkets. Students close their eyes and take an item, feeling it without looking.
k. *Touchstone* is any stone or pebble, kept in the pocket as a simple reminder to relax into awareness and smile.
l. *Formal Body Meditation* involves body awareness or scans for longer time periods, often found free online. Use the guidance above for these longer durations.

5. *See Moments*
   a. *Just See* the world around you and/or the world inside (of mental images, colors, or movies) without initiating thoughts about what is seen. Thoughts may come, but do not latch on to any such labeling, judging, or other mental commentary. Allow for the possibility of *becoming* seeing.
   b. *Intense Presence* arises from focusing as completely as possible on almost anything nearby (e.g., the bark of a tree, an open window) such that thoughts may drop away. If and when there is a cessation of thoughts, it may produce a shock of bliss, though it may take repeated practice to relax through not thinking.
   c. *Notice for the First Time* by becoming absorbed in a familiar object (e.g., desk, bed, wristwatch) with complete freshness by *not naming, not describing* or thinking at all, but seeing something as though for the first time.
   d. *See the Sky* encourages frequent, momentary glances upward at whatever slice of sky may be viewable, taking inside the vastness and beauty of what is there.
   e. *Eyes of Love* is to look at anyone (new or familiar) without any mental description or labeling, just taking in the person with love and acceptance. Notice how this impacts social interactions and well-being (see *gazing*, p. 245 for more).
   f. *Near, Far, and All* is a silent viewing journey starting with (1) seeing the tip of the nose then (2) looking into the most distant point viewable, then (3) focusing on the space halfway between and then (4) extending the gaze and awareness in a 360-degree sphere around, above, behind, and below.
6. *Hear Moments*
   a. *Just Hear* the world around you and/or the world inside (of mental sounds, voices, or music) without initiating thoughts about what is heard. Thoughts may come, but do not latch on to any such labeling, judging, or other

mental commentary. Allow for the possibility of *becoming* hearing.
  b. *Tone Down* invites students to close their eyes and focus on a chime, bell, or any neutral tone that diminishes slowly over time (many are available on phones or apps). Students can take note when they don't hear anything and listen to silence.
  c. *X-Ray Ears* listen not just for the words being spoken by another but the meaning between them and the feelings behind them, all without any thought of replying.
  d. *Listen to Silence* is to patiently attune to gaps in sound, and if there is a steady sound, to listen for the silence beyond all sound.
7. Emotion Moments
  a. *Calm Place* can be imaginary or real, wherever one feels at ease. Picture the calm place and go there mentally, noting the sights, sounds, smells and more. Use this refuge whenever needed, or see "Taking Refuge" for more, p. 17.
  b. *Feeling Cue* is using a particular emotion (such as anger) as a cue (whenever it happens to be there) to mindfully pause, feel the emotion fully, and allow it to go, flow, or stay wherever it is in the body. Finish with a self-loving affirmation that acknowledges the achievement of emotional recognition in the moment.
  c. *Cherish Other* is relating with the knowledge that *this particular interaction* will never happen again. Invite this recognition to infuse any connection with preciousness, gratitude, and curiosity and see what unfolds.
  d. *Becoming the Pulse* is feeling the heartbeat, whether on the side of the neck, or inside the wrist, or over the heart, and attuning to whatever is being felt emotionally, or just sinking into the pulse itself with a soft warmth to self.
  e. *Phone Feels* are sensed progressively by noting feelings about a personal device without putting any energy into thoughts. Progress through each phase for a few seconds

starting with (1) the phone turned off and placed in front of you, then (2) picking up the turned-off device, and (3) turning it on but not touching it.
   f. *Receiving Vibes* is to open up and deeply sense the next person you see, noticing their "feeling tone" or vibe, without judgment and then letting it go.
8. *Mixed Moments*
   a. *Just Do It* makes the mundane magical by doing anything routine (e.g., driving a familiar route, filling a water bottle, brushing teeth, or pulling back a chair) with absolute presence. Routine tasks are often done with a haze of distracted thinking but "just do it" is the opposite: complete absorption, potentially transforming the task into a vivid, engaged experience of life. Choose seomthing simple to start and then incorporate other tasks. Debrief often to refresh this rewarding practice and share any insights or discoveries.
   b. *Mindful Talking* uses no *ums*, *ers*, or *ahs* in speech, just pure presence in speaking deepest truths—easy to describe but hard to do.
   c. *Skin Breathing* imagines breath flowing in and out through the entire surface of the body, simultaneously activating body and breath awareness.
   d. *Auto-Mindfulness* can be used by drivers and passengers alike.
      i. *Stop sign*: stop completely and take a breath.
      ii. *Red light*: interrupt any incessant thinking and see the red light as warming your heart.
      iii. *Yield*: when that next person wants in, let them in and wish them well.
      iv. *Speed limit sign*: check your speed, in the car and in life. Decide if it feels good and adjust if needed; usually slower feels better.
   e. *Walking Mindfulness* is to walk as though on sacred ground, taking every step with reverence and absolute

presence. Notice the multiple sensations of balance and weight, breathing and all, with warmth and acceptance.

f. *Openings to Presence* could be a door to a room, a car door, or opening of any kind. When moving through such portals, use that moment to come back to a relaxed awareness of life, letting go of what you don't need and leaving it at the door.

g. *Crossing the Streams* involves a progressive scan of the "just feel," "just see," and "just hear" streams of awareness described above, noticing each without judgment. One can linger in a particular stream, cross them all in succession, or let them mix and possibly become aware of all of them together. These three streams can become six if there is a discernment between inner and outer experience, such as noticing mental images or movies versus what is seen in the outside world.

h. *Labeling* thoughts as they appear can help prevent getting lost in them and provide some distance from thinking. A label could be "imagining," "remembering," "worrying," "planning," or simply "helpful" or "unhelpful." Let the thought(s) come and go, welcoming them all. Also see *self-directed neuroplasticity* (p. 156).

i. *Become*, even for just a moment, a bird, baby, flower, gust of wind, or any phenomena that is pleasing. Take the shape, sound, and feel of it with your body, voice, and heart, letting go of everything else. Relish in being anything.

j. *Clock Watching* has students pair up to take turns watching the second hand of a clock for two (or more) minutes. While partner A watches the clock, they indicate lapses in concentration by lifting a finger, and total concentration derailments by raising their whole hand, going back to clock watching each time. Partner B quietly watches partner A do this. Time the experience, and switch roles without any discussion. Debrief (see p. 16) after both have had a turn, and then debrief as a whole class, particularly getting at self-compassion for lapses. Repeat with the

instruction to watch the clock *lovingly*, as though it was a child being cared for, and see if that makes any difference.
    k. *Accept All* is an invitation to consider the possibility of *completely accepting everything* in life: all people, situations, personal challenges—everything. Acceptance does not imply complacency but merely a peacefulness of not resisting reality, and then facing and living that reality.
    l. *5-4-3-2-1* is a sequence of sensing starting with the eyes open taking in *five* things you can see, then closing the eyes and noting *four* sounds, then *three* touch sensations, *two* smells/tastes and *one* emotion.
9. *Debrief*: Celebrate insights and changes by debriefing mindful moments often, especially those used frequently. While positive qualities felt in a mindful moment may be fleeting, with practice they may linger and grow into persistent wellness qualities. This critical growth aspect of the practice can be highlighted in the debriefs.
10. *Integration Strategy*: Use mindful moments in the context of daily classroom life
    - to prepare students at the beginning of learning;
    - in transitions between activities, or as natural breaks in a period, day, or unit; and
    - as a calming finish to end learning.
11. *Lifeplay*: Mindful moments are a natural to use throughout daily life beyond school—including at home. Effectiveness relies on frequent use, so encourage lifeplay, solicit student experiences, and model by sharing your own teacher lifeplay stories.
12. *Schoolwide Extension*: Use these moments with teams, clubs, staff meetings, or during assemblies to share the practices widely and build a school culture of calm awareness.

Keywords: card, caring, cognitive, choice, emotional, eudaimonia, foundational, gratitude, hedonia, icebreaker, integration, lifeplay, mindfulness, outdoor, prep-free, resilience, schoolwide, social, short-'n'-safe, spiritual

Self-Directed Neuroplasticity (Main Move)

> "The truly important manifestation of will, the one from which our decisions and behaviors flow, is the choice we make about the quality and direction of attentional focus. Mindful or unmindful, wise or unwise—no choice we make is more basic, or important, than this one."[12]
>
> —Jeffrey M. Schwartz

Our mental travels are often circular, so a small tilt up or down can make all the difference. After getting 32 percent on his first physics quiz, Luka has a cognitive train wreck: not only will he fail the course—and all of school—but he *himself* is a failure, with no chance for redemption. His teacher Ms. Moussa has been assigned physics for the first time and is feeling like a bit of an imposter, at first. She keeps focusing on adapting positively and has reached out to another physics teacher in the district for support. Her habit is to see struggle as emblematic of courage and resilience, which is why she was given this new opportunity in the first place.

Both Luka and Ms. Moussa have woven a mental pattern by habit—one harmful, one helpful—which literally changes their brain. This incredible capacity for *self-directed neuroplasticity* arises from several key qualities.

- *Will*: our human capacity to choose and maintain attentional focus
- *Plasticity*: the brain's changeability throughout life, not just in youth
- *Association*: the tendency for neurons that fire together to wire together
- *Patterning*: the streamlining and strengthening of mental patterns through repetition
- *Decay*: the diminishing of inactive neural connections

These qualities combine to rewire the brain for wellness over time through repeated, non-invasive, brain "operations." These operations can flexibly groove positivity or mitigate a host of cognitive challenges like stress, anxiety, depression, bias, addiction, or even the brain's own inherent negativity bias.[13] Months after practicing self-directed neuroplasticity, significant increases in positive emotions persist, while negative emotions decrease.[14]

On the positive side of self-directed neuroplasticity, "savoring" involves noticing, intensifying, and integrating good experiences. These experiences could be happy memories, the anticipation of future goodness, or a healthy focus on what's good right now. On the side of negative experiences, self-directed neuroplasticity can downregulate negativity, pivot thinking upward, or engage in the crucial—and cognitively purifying—practice of complete acceptance. Rewiring negativity can boost well-being even more than savoring, especially where a negativity bias is strong.[15] The activity below suggests a positive practice with which to begin and then several options to work with negativity using the same core operations.

Self-directed neuroplasticity benefits also extend to other wellness domains beyond the cognitive, boosting physical health, emotional regulation, and eudaimonic self-determination. Sharing what's good with others, and asking about their goodness, capitalizes socially on cognitive practice.[16]

In a world of immediate gratification, students and teachers can learn to appreciate the long-term empowerment that comes from self-directed neuroplasticity. Habitual cultivation of healthy thinking becomes a lasting trait that tilts the spiral of mental activity upward.

> **Summary**: Rewire one's own mind for wellness with repeated neural "operations."
> **Time**: 10 minutes (initial), 10–30 seconds (ongoing)
> **Trust Required**: Low-medium
>
> 0. *Teach Neuroscience* (5 minutes): Facilitate some basic learning around brain science to boost interest and acceptance, especially if there is a curricular connection, and perhaps using some of the citations given. At minimum, convey that self-directed neuroplasticity is training one's own thoughts (mind) to rewire the brain. These three "CORE" steps to "RECUPERATE" cognitive well-being are easy to remember:[17]
>   a. *cue* (an event which initiates a mental operation);

b. *operate* (doing the self-directed neuroplasticity operation itself); and
   c. *repeat* (repetition makes new patterns over time, tilting the mental spiral up).
1. *Cue* (1 minute): Create some anticipation by telling students you will share a self-directed neuroplasticity practice when the right moment cues it. Put a question mark on the board to represent this mysterious moment. The cue in this practice (joy farming) is any positive experience, individual or shared. In the classroom, this could be a joke that cracks everyone up, or singing happy birthday. When this happens, point out the positive cue and proceed to step 2. Later, as this practice builds, students and teachers can find and use a wide variety of positive experiences as a cue:
   a. anything positive in the present moment: a shared donut or sunlight streaming;
   b. remembering good memories of the past;
   c. anticipating good things to come in the future;
   d. feeling gratitude for a bed, clean water, or loved ones;
   e. luxuriating in the pleasure of a hot shower, luscious chocolate, or fun game;
   f. marveling at beauty in nature, art, or anything awesome;
   g. elevation in witnessing inspiring acts (see p. 66); and/or
   h. basking in pride after getting praise, loving oneself, or any accomplishment.
2. *Operate* (2 minutes): Invite the class to "FARM" the joy and goodness in the immediate aftermath of the positive experience by leading them through these steps:[18]
   a. *Focus* fully by putting complete attention on the emotions, body senses, or thoughts arising from the experience to intensify and immerse oneself in it. Physical postures, such as spreading arms like wings to mimic a bird in flight, or smiling broadly, may help in deeply *becoming* the experience.

b. *Associate* the experience with other memories—noting what is new, different, or meaningful about it—to help make stronger neural connections.

c. *Remain* in the experience, even after the event itself has passed, for 5 seconds, 15 seconds, 30 seconds, or more to increase brain wiring time.

d. *Marinate* in it all, letting all the goodness permeate, sink in, and wire the brain. Use a visualization, like warm light, or just let it happen naturally.

3. *Repeat* (1 minute × repetitions): Frequency of practice is the surest way to lasting change. While long-term memory is aided by association or strong emotions, these are not always available, so repeat, repeat, repeat. The following strategies can aid repetition:

   a. *In-class*: continue to notice and harvest good experiences, repeating steps 1 and 2, but reducing guidance as students learn. Jot down each experience on the board, and be sure to participate as a teacher to keep the practice going.

   b. *Lifeplay*: using self-directed neuroplasticity throughout life outside school is a no-brainer (and grow-brainer) for establishing healthy thoughts in the long term. See "Using Life to Free Yourself" (p. 123) for more cueing ideas.

   c. *Debrief*: use the standard debrief (see p. 16) from time to time to resurface the practice. Discuss any changes or other observations to reactivate the steps and celebrate progress made.

4. *Working with Negativity*: Harmful or unhelpful thoughts can also be cues to retrain the brain, whether in school or out. Table 6.1 offers several ways to do this using the same "CORE" steps as the joy farming above. In this way, negative thought loops become opportunities to wire in more positive patterns. Adding a positive twist to a negative experience is not always required. Just noticing harmful thoughts and stopping their momentum can help. As thinking tilts upward,

negative cues will occur less often. The most vital step—repeat—is shown for emphasis.
5. *Safety*: Positive effects may be reduced if there is excessive comparison: such as with other people's lives, a peak event from the past (which may never happen again), or a feeling that something better *should* have happened. Encourage students to be selective about which experiences will genuinely feel positive to them, whether past, present, or future. There are choices about which practices feel good, so encourage the dropping of practices that don't seem to help, and take a break or try something else. See also "Taking Refuge" safety considerations (p. 21).
6. *Integration Strategy*: Watch for opportunities amid learning topics where students may use self-directed neuroplasticity to either
   a. savor a positive moment such as learning a tough concept or skill;
   b. work with negative self-talk such as "I can't do this"; and/or
   c. absorb a particular curricular concept or skill by holding it in mind.

Keywords: caring, cognitive, choice, emotional, empower, foundational, gratitude, hedonia, integration, lifeplay, mindfulness, prep-free, resilience, short-'n'-safe, support

COGNITIVE WELL-BEING

Table 6.1. Self-Directed Neuroplasticity CORE Steps

Practice	<u>C</u>ue	<u>O</u>perate	<u>Re</u>peat
Joy Farming	(See 1 above)	(See 2 above)	(See 3 above)
Coming Alongside	Any challenging or stressful thought or experience.	Come alongside the experience, relaxing into any sensations without fueling them, just feeling them. Come alongside self, generating warmth and kindness for oneself.	(See 3 above)
Useful or Not?	Unhelpful thoughts, particularly thoughts that resurface incessantly, or noticing a habit that is harmful rather than helpful. Example: excessive worry, perhaps about an upcoming assignment due date.	Label the thought "useful" if it helps in some way. Example: Useful. I haven't started. I'll get to work now. Label the thought "not useful" if it doesn't help. Move on. Example: Not useful, I've already submitted it, and I did my best. Good for me.	(See 3 above)
True or Not? (Belief Testing)	Partially or completely false or exaggerated thoughts, about oneself or others. Cognitive distortions, such as catastrophic thinking, personalizing, magnifying, minimizing or mindreading make excellent cues here. Example: Nobody ever shows up to class on time, they just don't care about me.	Ask "Is this thought true?" and sometimes "Is this thought absolutely, always true?" to counter unrealistic or extreme thinking. Consider what positive aspects are true or could be true. Example: Most students do arrive on time on most days. Maja said good morning to me.	(See 3 above)

Table 6.1. *(continued)*

Practice	<u>C</u>ue	<u>O</u>perate	<u>R</u>epeat
Reshaping, Reframing, Redirecting	Unuseful or untrue thoughts (see above) that include an element of negativity such as anxiety or negative self-talk. *Example: I'm so stupid.*	Savor something positive that counters or softens the negativity. *Example: I helped Luka figure out his new phone pretty quickly. I'm good at that.*	(See 3 above)
Labeling	Any thought, feeling, or even body sensation can be a cue for labeling. Labeling thoughts can lessen the "stickiness" of thinking. Practice for a few minutes at a time or as long as it feels helpful.	Mentally label or softly speak whatever thought or feeling is there. *Example: "future," "planning," "satisfaction," "remembering," "worry," "assumption," "shiver," etc.*	(See 3 above)
Ceasing	Any negative, unhelpful thought loops or patterns.	Just saying no to the thought. Staying very present, so as to not feed the cycle of negative thinking can be a relief.	(See 3 above)
Wise and Loving Mind	Any dilemma, decision, or problem, especially where there is a stuck feeling.	Ask "What would a wise, loving person/friend say?" This person/friend could be real or imagined.	(See 3 above)
Three Filters	Any thought that doesn't pass the three filters of being true, necessary, and kind.	Think of what is actually true, necessary, or kind. If that's nothing, move on gracefully.	(See 3 above)

From Semi-Interested to Flow: Games and Experiments in Immersive States

> "The best moments in our lives are not the passive, receptive, relaxing times—although such experiences can also be enjoyable, if we have worked hard to attain them. The best moments usually occur when a person's body or mind is stretched to its limits in a voluntary effort to accomplish something difficult and worthwhile."[19]
>
> —Mihaly Csikszentmihalyi

Dakota liked physics class—a lot. Mr. Charles was a solid teacher, told corny jokes, and always gave tests back the day after they were written. He could also draw perfect circles freehand, which delighted Dakota to no end. But what Dakota loved most was practicing for the physics olympiad after school. When she dove into the practice contests, her entire world became the problem on the page. In her mind, quantities, unknowns, and formulae rearranged themselves effortlessly to squeeze out the solutions. In those times, she wasn't aware of Mr. Charles helping others, or even herself, and when practice ended, she would look up and realize she had to pee.

Students like Dakota are every teacher's dream: immersed in learning, working at peak while improving that peak, and feeling fulfilled. Most teachers would love to feel this way in their own work from time to time. Being completely "in the zone" feels like being carried blissfully downstream, hence the term *flow*. Immersive states of all depths can boost learning and well-being, from the optimal experience of flow right on down to lesser states of engagement.

On this point, there's no need to be snobbish about peak experiences. Most teachers would welcome even a smidgen of engagement in students, if not total flow. Deep states such as Dakota's are wonderful, but wellness can arise from a broad spectrum of immersion, whether students are semi-interested, engaged, or totally absorbed:[20]

- Groups work math problems at stand-up whiteboards with a noisy engagement, while the teacher circulates to add or remove challenges for each group.
- A science class is captivated watching a time-lapse video.

- A language student becomes engrossed in reading a personally chosen book.
- Two students edit a video interview with rapt concentration to meet a deadline in a communication technology class.
- A geography class is immersed in a test for which they have been well prepared.
- A senior trumpet player is lost in a solo at an end-of-term music performance exam.
- Two badminton team members are in the total flow of an epic, extended rally during practice, watched with pin-drop enthrallment by teammates.

The deepest flow states are rare, but can produce a defining experience of transcendence, a key aspect of the spiritual domain. This highlights again the interconnectedness of well-being. As awareness of self diminishes in a flow task, there is a *merging* of awareness and task, providing some profound and powerful well-being benefits:

- complete absence of day-to-day problems or anxiety;
- elimination of self-oriented thought, or even any conscious thought;
- a diminished or lost sense of time; and/or
- effortlessness—a feeling of abundant energy.

Additional wellness benefits of immersive states can be found in the cognitive domain (through engagement and joy), eudaimonic domain (in fulfillment and growth), and emotional domain (from heightened emotional regulation).[21] Indeed, the many wonders of flow have spurred humanity's development of the arts, physical sports, and most every hobby under the sun. Creating a flow-tacular classroom opens the door for youth to experience such immersive states, with their corresponding well-being benefits. Teachers also benefit from the challenge, engagement, and fulfillment of helping young people get there.

As wonderful as flow feels, when an activity lacks or loses meaning, the pleasure can fade. Similarly, and intense and/or prolonged focus on a minor aspect of life may negatively impact overall wellness. Healthy flourishing is sustained from activities in a variety of well-being domains, and a range of immersive states—not just peak experience. Learning to move from an empty habit or small detail to something more substantial is a skill grounded in intuition, discipline, and self-love.

After a long week teaching grade 7 students, Ryan would grab some food and start gaming. With his penchant for fantasy, the virtual world was a rich escape. The dozens of hours he spent improving skills and completing achievements—motivated by addictive game rewards—only deepened his immersion. The tougher challenges felt best: a sweet spot of complex problem solving. Ryan rarely felt this way in the classroom, and he also knew he'd been neglecting teaching of late.

After spending hours grinding for a small in-game perk, Ryan felt hollow. Playing no longer satisfied him, it only reminded him of what he was avoiding. He shut down his console and turned to a stack of neglected student writing. Digging in, he wondered if there were ways to make writing assignments as engaging as gaming. He fell into a rhythm of reading, writing feedback, and making notes for the next unit based on student interests. He soon began to feel absorbed again, but this time in a good way.

Mihaly Csikszentmihalyi, the progenitor of flow, describes the power inherent in fusing the immersive with the meaningful: "A person who has achieved control over psychic energy and has invested it in consciously chosen goals cannot help but grow into a more complex being. By stretching skills, by reaching toward higher challenges, such a person becomes an increasingly extraordinary individual." Experiments by Csikszentmihalyi and others have revealed conditions, catalysts, and indicators for flow.[22]

This activity invites teachers to get interested and actively involved with these parameters, making changes to the learning environment, instructional strategies, tasks, and feedback in the interest of producing classroom flow. While there are no silver bullets that guarantee immersion, making a game and an experiment out of adjusting these parameters might engage a few students, while helping teachers discover some flow for themselves in the process.

Table 6.2. Conditions, Catalysts, and Indicators of Immersive Flow in the Classroom

Conditions	Catalysts	Indicators
• Challenging tasks that match the skill level of the doer. • "Goldilocks" tasks that aren't too hard, but aren't too easy. • Tasks that match personal interests, skills, or desires.	• Skill-building before significant tasks. • Scaffolding tasks to reduce challenge, or extensions that increase challenge, according to student readiness. • Differentiating for (and providing student choice in) all aspects of a task: topics, processes, products, and assessment (see p. 26). • Applying and connecting learning to what is relevant and real for students, revealing a task's *meaning*.	• Neither a feeling of boredom nor anxiety, but somewhere in between. • Personal needs fade or disappear, such as the need for a break or to have lunch.
• A capacity to focus on the task at hand, with purity and intensity.	• Practicing mindfulness (see p. 145) to increase concentration skills. • Reducing excessive thinking with some physical activity. • Creating a quiet, safer environment that minimizes distractions. • Silencing or removing technology. • Giving students time and coaching, to help them take care of responsibilities and other commitments.	• A magical silence, or focused bustle that descends on the classroom when students are deeply engaged.
• Clear goals with immediate, ongoing feedback.	• Use online simulations or gamified learning tools with clear objectives and ongoing, in-the-moment feedback. • Provide success criteria up front, in student-friendly language, for ongoing self-assessment (see p. 110). • Allowing multiple opportunities.	• Feelings of reward and enjoyment, even for challenging tasks, or where the task is incomplete.
• Automatic, spontaneous actions that merge with awareness.	• Allowing significant time for the grooving of skills to develop automaticity. • Noticing and celebrating when any classroom skill is shown to have been deeply assimilated.	• Capacity for students to use ingrained skills in unfamiliar and complex contexts.
• A sense of influence, agency, or control over what's happening.	• Reducing or eliminating competition, especially where the competition overshadows the activity itself.	• A feeling of confidence, but also with the sense that growth is happening.
• For group efforts, a diminishment of individual needs in favor of group cohesion, and strong inter-group relationships.	• Consider removing grades entirely (but not feedback), especially where it sets up students for competition or discourages groupthink. • Develop strong student-student relationships (see social well-being, p. 55).	• Feelings of fulfillment doing the experience, for its own sake.

Summary: Experiment with classroom factors that make immersive states more likely.
Time: Varies
Trust Required: Low

1. *Introduction* (15 minutes): Play a short video, or give a short lesson, on the concept of flow or immersive states, and hold a class discussion. Project or display table 6.2.
   a. Invite students to share experiences of flow from their lives, including the arts, exercise, play, sports, games, hobbies, or any experience that produced immersive qualities. Draw out their descriptions of flow experiences, along with aspects of the situation or task (see table 6.2) that brought on immersion.
   b. Encourage students to watch for, and report back to the class, any flow experiences they have, whether in school or out. They can begin noticing these in areas of personal interest or aptitude (see "Lifeplay" below).
2. *Integration Strategy* (varies): Teachers use table 6.2 to review and implement some of the catalysts (column 2) in their lesson planning, focusing on tasks that meet more of the conditions (column 1). For example, teachers could modify an assignment to be student self-assessed and give multiple opportunities for feedback cycles. Or teachers could give more differentiation options, making it more likely for students to reach an optimal level of challenge.
3. *Lifeplay* (varies): Encourage students to look for flow in activities where it would not usually arise, such as the daily tasks of school or family life. While it's easier to get immersed in gaming or enjoyable sports, becoming more engaged is possible in every task of life, no matter how mundane. For example, in cutting grass, practicing a deep task focus (keeping the mower on the edge), then finding some kind of challenge

in that task (covering the area in as few passes as possible) hones skill and increases absorption.
4. *Debrief* (varies): Seek student feedback on any immersive experiences that may be happening in or out of class. Explore both the nature of the experience (however deep or shallow) and any factors that contributed to it. Point out any efforts made to stay "in the zone" in class. This could be putting on headphones to tune out noise, asking for help to begin a task, or making a game out of doing homework questions as quickly and accurately as possible with a seatmate.
5. *Safety*: Some activities are more conducive to flow due to their inherent challenge (e.g., rock climbing), but safety must always be considered before engaging in the task.

Keywords: cognitive, choice, creative, eudaimonia, hedonia, integration, lifeplay, mindfulness, physical

Train That Train

Is your train of thoughts a train wreck or a gravy train? Helping yourself and others to become aware of mental self-talk is a significant step forward on the path of cognitive awareness and well-being. In seeing the tracks of our thought patterns we can train our mind toward a wholesome destination.

Summary: Write down a stream of thoughts and reflect on it personally, with compassion.
Time: 10 minutes
Trust Required: Low

1. *Write* (3 minutes): Invite students to write down their thoughts as they arise, without trying to think about anything in particular, for three minutes. Reassure them that whatever is written will not be shared, as it is for private reflection only.

At the end of the time ask them to pause and take a few moments of silence and gratitude for having the awareness to do such an activity. As always, the teacher participates in the activity with the students while facilitating, both to better appreciate the experience as well as to personally benefit.

2. *Reflect* (2 minutes): Students and teacher individually review their written thoughts using the following annotation symbols. Encourage a kind-hearted, accepting attitude.
    a. Note "+" (plus sign) beside positive or useful thoughts and "–" for negative or unhelpful thoughts.
    b. Jot "P" beside thoughts of the past, "F" for future and "N" for now.
    c. Write "X" beside unreal or untrue thoughts, and "✓" beside true ones.
    d. Put a "?" near extreme or judgmental thoughts, which may include words like "always," "everybody," "totally," "never," "should," "must," or "have to."
    e. Use "!" for any thought that stands out in some way.
    f. Put "♡" beside loving or kind thoughts about others and "♡♡" for self-love.

3. *Debrief* (5 minutes): Seek reflections on the writing process itself, and then whatever people most noticed, inviting some whole-group sharing with these prompts:
    a. Does writing out your thoughts change your perspective on them?
    b. The brain is a brilliant and beautiful organ capable of creativity, imagination, problem solving and so much more. How do our thoughts serve us—or not? What do they tell us or suggest?
    c. Is it possible to train these trains of thought by choosing or changing to different ones? What can we do about unhelpful or negative thoughts? (See *self-directed neuroplasticity* on p. 156 for strategies to do this.)

4. *Safety*: The process of writing automatically provides some distance from thoughts, making the activity a safer way to

explore mental tendencies. Ensure anonymity by having students keep and/or destroy their recorded thoughts after the activity.
5. *Integration Strategy*: Students can write about a curriculum topic, and also their *feelings* about the topic, and look for a judgmental or supportive stance toward their learning.
6. *Lifeplay*: Where students keep personal journals, invite them to add a layer of reflection on the thoughts, similar to what is described above.

Keywords: caring, cognitive, integration, journal, mindfulness, prep-free, resilience, short-'n'-safe, support

SUPPLEMENTARIES: SHORT, SIMPLE, SAFE, OR SEARCHABLE COGNITIVE WELL-BEING

- *Brain Breaks* could be almost anything: pencil flipping tricks, making a wave in the class, dances, puzzles, games, or just turning the desks backward. Variety and surprise make a break that much fresher, so consider letting students choose and lead breaks to keep things fresh.[23] *Search terms*: brain breaks, [high school], [middle school].
- *Cognitive Distortion Scavenger Hunt* is a cheeky game played in two stages. In stage 1, students pair up to research a single cognitive distortion such as catastrophizing, emotional reasoning, or the fallacy of fairness. These are shared with the class, along with an example for each. By the end, students will have a list of ten or fifteen cognitive distortions. In stage 2, they carry their list with them, watching for these behaviors in themselves or others. (This can be done in class only and/or as lifeplay.) Students do not point out the distortions in others but simply notice. Debrief after two weeks to see which distortions were found and whether being aware of them has changed cognitive well-being in any way. *Search terms*: cognitive distortions.

- *Coloring Hath Charms* to soothe the anxious student or teacher.[24] Immersion in the mindful coloring of a mandala or natural scene may reduce anxiety and provide a pleasant flow experience. *Search terms*: mindful, coloring, mandala [image search].
- *Connect the Dots* makes explicit links between what students are learning with: prior learning, other subjects, their own lives, and the world at large. Application makes concepts meaningful and memorable. The brain is made of neural connections, and so it feels good to make more of them this way. *Search terms*: making, learning, connections.
- *Creativity Is Joy* affirms the link between happiness and creative pursuits by immersing in almost any life activity with originality and personal expression. Painting, writing, or dancing are obvious options, but take up the challenge of finding creativity in cooking, gardening, speaking, or giving a hug. *Search terms*: creativity, happiness, joy.
- *Decision Time* is the gift of 5 minutes of classroom time, perhaps weekly or daily, for basic life planning and prioritizing. Students and teachers ease their cognitive loads by getting out phone calendars or agendas and planning for various responsibilities. Invite sharing around what organizational strategies work for different people.[25] Be sure to discuss the caretaking of responsibilities and commitments explicitly:
  - What prioritization or management strategies do students use (if any)?
  - How does it feel to take care of things—or let them slide? What is the impact of these decisions on the rest of our lives?
  - How can we develop the skill of organization in our classroom together?
- *Learning Circles* add the social-emotional benefits of circle work to learning, whether at the beginning, middle, or end of a learning cycle. Both whole-class or small-group learning circles run much like check-in circles (p. 57). Students can share learning with classmates and get feedback or do presentations in a circle. Curriculum-based thumballs (p. 80) enhance learning circles. Experiment and discover what works best for your subject, starting with these learning circle prompts:

- "What is your prior knowledge about . . . ?"
- "What do you hope to explore or learn about . . . ?"
- "What concerns you about this topic, and what would help you?"
- "Share your (project, essay, or assignment) topic for feedback regarding . . ."
- "What connections can you make between . . . ?"
- "Reflecting on the learning in this unit, book, topic, what do you think about . . . ?"
- "What are you still wondering or have questions about . . . ?"
- "What have you best learned about . . . ?"
- "My strengths and challenges with this subject, topic, unit, . . ."
- "What helps me most in learning . . ."

- *Mental Health and Mindfulness Apps* abound, and have a variety of features, but classes can start with well-developed apps that are free for education such as Calm, Headspace, Insight Timer, or Stop, Breathe and Think. *Search terms:* teenage, youth, app [mental health, mindfulness]
- *Plantastic* considers how well-organized your lesson, unit, or course truly is, and whether plans get shared with the class ahead of time. Involve students to get feedback and ideas. When school feels "plantastic" both student and teacher mental stress evaporates.
- *Thought Journaling* consists of journal entries around thoughts and the situations in which they arise. Cognitive awareness and objectivity are cultivated through deciding which thoughts are most relevant and reflecting on them with equanimity.
- *Value Lines* flex mental views on any question or topic with a range of class opinions. Students line up physically from one end of the classroom (representing strongly disagree) to the other end (strongly agree). Fold the line to make pairs, or form heterogeneous groups taken from every part of the line to start a discussion. After some discussion, students can reform another line, encouraging participants to *change their position*. Highlight anyone who changes views and ask why they did so. Repeat the process if it serves. Wellness arises from sharing divergent views respectfully, listening to different perspectives, and considering whether one's own mental positions can shift. An alternative to a lineup is to use four corners of the room.

- *Watched Words* recognizes the power words have over thoughts and well-being. Reality-rejecting words like *should, shouldn't, have to, must,* or *need to* may create non-acceptance and judgment. Phrases including these words typically reinforce their inherent negativity. Extreme words like *never, always, everyone, nobody, everywhere,* and *nowhere* can reinforce cognitive distortions such as maximizing and catastrophizing. Invite students to watch for these words in their speech and come up with alternatives. Debrief the impact of using alternatives, and if so, how they feel. Some alternatives to watched words are provided here (also see "Resili-entences," p. 139):
    - "I should work out more" could become "I feel great when I work out."
    - "You shouldn't be talking during my lesson" could become "It's difficult for me and others when you talk during my lesson."
    - "I shouldn't be feeling sad" could become "I'm feeling sad because . . . "
    - "I never get anything right" could become "I get a few things right."
    - "Everyone is wasting time today" could become "Neli and Blake, get to work."
- *Wiser Students, Wiser World* is a call for teachers to incorporate information literacy, media literacy, and scientific literacy into their programs. Identifying bias, understanding context, detecting fake news (or junk science), thinking critically, and using trustworthy sources of evidence-based information are key skills for students to be healthy themselves, and to create a healthy world. These emerging literacies can be readily integrated into almost any subject, and have powerful impacts for the well-being of future generations. *Search terms*: teaching, students, information literacy, media literacy, scientific literacy

7

EMOTIONAL WELL-BEING

Hedonia and Beyond

"Without our emotions, we can't make decisions; we can't decipher our dreams and visions; we can't set proper boundaries or behave skillfully in relationships; we can't identify our hopes or support the hopes of others; and we can't connect to, or even find, our dearest loves."[1]

—Karla McLaren

Decades of computer science in schools have resulted in 30 billion devices on the internet, exchanging data worldwide. Modern science education, which began in the mid-nineteenth century, has produced colliders that smash particles with unfathomable energies, confirming the standard model of physics. Apprenticeships in technology and the teaching of mathematics have been a part of formal learning for centuries, and now telescopes in space can see ten thousand galaxies in a pinhead of sky stretching back 13 billion years.

It's miraculous to consider that some teachers today have been alive for the dawn of the information age, the unveiling of the universe, and the splitting of the heart of matter itself. Yet for all these monumental achievements, we have only the faintest inkling of our own human hearts. Our greatest social institutions have largely failed to explicitly teach the language, inner workings, and wonder of emotions. The impact of this oversight is staggering and tragic.

Emotional underdevelopment has contributed to countless wars, famines, genocides, slavery, and other atrocities. Our failure to intentionally develop empathy, self-compassion, or even to regulate base instincts, factors into abuse, neglect, poverty, social injustice, and environmental devastation. The same emotional dysfunction at the root of this incalculable harm also inhibits the very healing of the trauma it has left behind.

Humans are a wondrous paradox: big-brained, yet often unaware of our emotional core. A turbocharged digital age and overclocked social media have only widened this mind-heart chasm.[2] Education hasn't helped much, focusing on academics and leaving emotional development to families or extracurriculars. While some young people may get positive emotional modeling in their families, others live in unhealthy homes that undermine well-being.

Joshua's grade-10 English class had many students from such homes. These challenges, combined with some student-student friction had made disrespect and disruption the norm in his classroom. Any classroom management strategies he tried only seemed to make things worse. In desperation, he invited the school social worker to observe his class and help if possible. When she arrived, some students shut down with a new adult in the room, but others acted out even more. As the two staff moved to deal with each disturbance, another popped up across the room.

After twenty minutes, the social worker politely asked the student she was with to excuse her, pushed back her chair with a loud scrape, and stood up. Every head turned, and the room went quiet. Visibly upset, but breathing evenly, she did something nobody had tried: expressing authentic feelings with total sincerity. "I feel *drained* and . . . *sad* being here today. I can't know what it's like for all of you, but I'm feeling so frustrated being here. Is this how you really want it to be?" The defiant tone in the room shifted ever-so-briefly to a fragile remorse. Joshua gazed about in wonder, daring only to smile inside so as not to break the spell. While the behavior didn't resolve entirely after that, it improved by an order of magnitude. It was a start.

Schools are also making a start with emotional development. Though school staff may be in unfamiliar pedagogical territory, a social-emotional learning (SEL) (r)evolution is underway:

- Interest in SEL has ramped up since 2015, particularly in the United States, Singapore, Philippines, Australia, Canada, the United Kingdom, and Kenya.[3]
- In 2022, just over half of U.S. states are including SEL free-standing competencies in K-12, a 50 percent increase since 2020, with many adding guidance for implementation.[4]
- Pioneering schools and teachers are implementing SEL programs and training, not just in response to unwellness but to support efforts in equity, inclusion, and human rights.

There is much evidence to support these directions, as SEL develops emotional intelligence (EQ), which correlates powerfully to healthy relationships, academic achievement, positive work interactions, and well-being.[5] Even without an SEL program, teachers can have a profound impact by validating feelings and projecting a healthy positive, emotional field. Martin Seligman affirms these emotional efforts with his guiding hypothesis for positive education: "To the extent that teachers transmit optimism, trust, and a hopeful sense of the future, this will positively influence their students' perception of the world. . . . [P]ositive schools and positive teachers are the fulcrum for producing more well-being in a culture."[6]

But fulcrums need well-being too. Educator wellness is essential in its own right, and professional learning around emotional wellness helps staff and students alike. While teachers gain skills navigating the emotional maelstrom of pubescent students, they also come to understand and befriend their own feelings. Generations of youth can now benefit from an emotional education their own teachers, and their teachers' teachers, were denied.

HEDONIC ADAPTATION: FROM TREADMILL TO TRANSFORMATION

Despite a chaotic childhood in many schools, Andrea got straight As, went to teacher's college, and landed a job at a well-regarded school. Her success didn't come easily, and any joy Andrea felt for her accomplishments always seemed to go flat. After a work friend transferred to another school to become a vice principal, Andrea took on extra committee work and was promoted to department head. While the added responsibilities were permanent, the satisfaction was very temporary. Buying a new townhouse, taking trips abroad, and even two long-term relationships had left Andrea feeling like she was on a treadmill of seeking, comparing, and never feeling deeply fulfilled. She wondered if she would ever feel happy in a lasting way.

Andrea was indeed on a treadmill: a *hedonic treadmill*. This tendency for the brain to return to a neutral baseline state is also known as hedonic adaptation. Andrea's story relates to several findings around this phenomenon and the cultivation of emotional well-being:[7]

- About half of happiness is based on genetics: *what is given to us* through our ancestors. This is an estimate, but it's fair to say a good part of our emotional makeup is inherited.
- A much smaller slice of our happiness is due to life experiences: *what happens to us*. While happiness varies with experiences, it tends to return to a hedonic set point, though it takes longer to return after negative events because of the brain's negativity bias.
- Another large portion of our happiness—almost as much as genetics—is based on our self-determined, intentional thought and actions: *what we do with what happens to us*. In short, our baseline wellness is not fixed: we can change our level of happiness through conscious, willful actions.

This last point is vital for the emotional domain, or any other: *we can actively work to raise our well-being and keep it there over time*. We do this not just to overcome bad experiences but because we can lose sight of the good ones unless we find ways to refresh and keep them alive inside us. While this research is ever-evolving, it holds out hope that EQ can grow, and healthy emotional living can be both learned and taught.[8]

EQ is known as emotional intelligence, but actually stands for emotional quotient, inheriting a bias for all things mental from the term IQ. The emotional domain helps balance out this thinking obsession, but so too do skill-builders from other domains, including the cognitive. In fact, every other domain of well-being can contribute to emotional well-being. This rainbow of interconnections and activities are as important to explore as any activity in this chapter:

- sensing the inner body (*interoception,* p. 22) is an absolutely vital skill for detecting and discriminating emotional experience; be sure to use it in emotional wellness work;
- gratitude practices (p. 199) are an incredibly powerful counter to hedonic adaptation—refreshing what's good in life;
- mindfulness (p. 145) builds a stable platform to discern emotions, subtle or strong, as well as the serenity to be with emotional experience;
- response-ability practices (p. 115 and p. 123) are vital for managing strong emotions and making better responses in difficult moments;
- self-directed neuroplasticity (see p. 156) can work with emotions in a number of ways;
- the eudaimonic pursuit of what's meaningful and purposeful (see p. 85), not just pleasurable, and setting goals that transcend self (see p. 100) support long-term emotional well-being for oneself and everyone; and/or
- healthy, nourishing relationships (see p. 55) impact on emotional wellness enormously.

These skills take off when students have an emotional vocabulary to explore them. Growing a language of the heart in a safe environment gives expression to genuine feelings as skills are practiced. As emotional expression matures, EQ skills deepen, and so begins a positive feedback cycle of flourishing. As with the cognitive, emotional spirals can tilt upward.

Whether feelings go up or down, they run deep. And in those currents we can be swept to blissful peaks or over the abyss. But emotions color life; it is our human birthright and privilege to feel deeply. Teachers who can navigate these depths awaken students to the fullness of experience and enrich a magnificent domain of well-being that opens hearts to life and learning.

Key Messages

- Emotional development and well-being were traditionally left out of formal education, but they are now appearing in schools through social-emotional learning and other programs.
- Teacher emotional wellness is vital in its own right and helps with raising student EQ.
- Brains return to hedonic (happiness) setpoints after positive or negative experiences.
- Emotional wellness is largely inherited, but it can also be improved in lasting ways.
- Activities in multiple domains of well-being support emotional wellness and vice versa.

EMOTIONAL WELL-BEING ACTIVITIES

> "Some of you say, 'Joy is greater than sorrow,' and others say, 'Nay, sorrow is the greater.' But I say unto you, they are inseparable. Together they come, and when one sits alone with you at your board, remember that the other is asleep upon your bed."
>
> —Kalil Gibran

Feels Wheels (Main Move)

Having a language for emotional experience is fundamental for emotional literacy, expression, and empathy. *Feels Wheels* build a vocabulary of the heart, giving terminology for a wide range of nuanced feelings. Feels wheels are typically organized by emotional intensity and/or major emotional groupings using color, but a wide variety of different types are available. Find a wheel that has desirable features for you and your students.

- Robert Plutchik's wheel (see figure 7.1) places eight primary emotion groups across from their opposites and also shows combinations such as joy + anticipation = optimism.[9]
- The Junto wheel is a colorful, dense wheel of nuanced feelings in major sectors, along with a group dedicated to wonderful love.

EMOTIONAL WELL-BEING

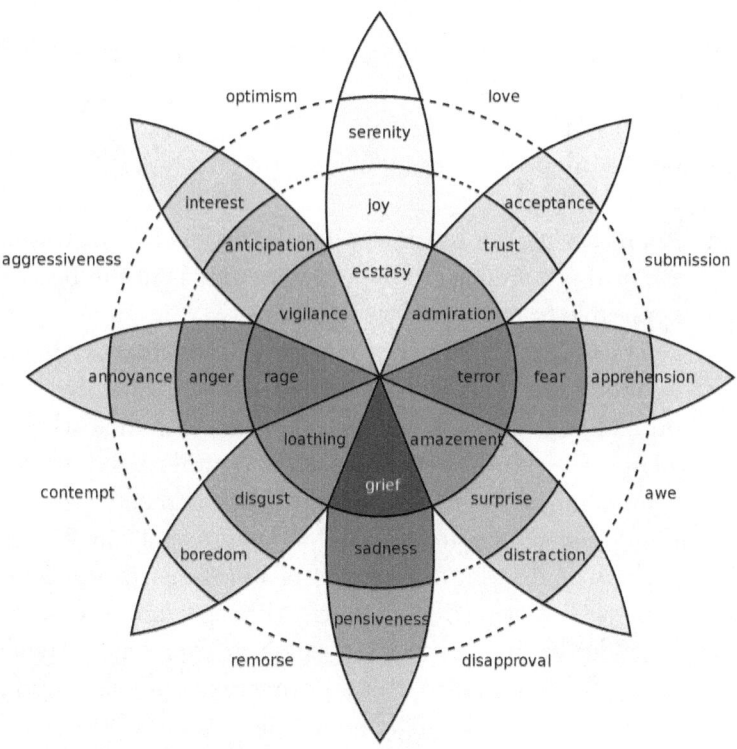

Figure 7.1. Plutchik Wheel of Emotions
Source: "Plutchik-Wheel", Wikimedia.org, February 12, 2011 (public domain).

- The Geneva wheel plots emotions along dimensions of pleasantness and control; it also includes a space for neutrality.
- Wheels with accompanying facial expressions or emojis (☺☺☺ ☺☺☺☺☺) provide pictorial cues to help students understand emotion words.

Feels wheels can be projected on screen during lessons and printed so each student has a personal reference. Teachers will also have their own copy, and it is vital for them to use it and share feelings along with the class. Consider feels wheels as a basic school supply to help students map their emotional world, voice their feelings, and understand others. Feels wheels can be used in a variety of ways as shown here, but also with most activities in this book, and with regular curricular work to help explore the emotional dimension of learning.

Summary: Develop emotional intelligence in a variety of ways using feels wheels.
Time: Varies
Trust Required: Low to medium

1. *Interoception* can be greatly aided using feels wheels (see p. 22) as it is a vital skill for sensing emotions in the body and applicable to many wellness domains.
2. *Check-in* with emotional words when students arrive to class, or after a weekend. Doing this regularly validates having and expressing feelings. Students can do this with their wheels in a circle check-in, by sticking pins in a poster-sized wheel, or completing an online survey to preserve anonymity.
3. *Emoji and Expression* invites students to put emojis (using stickers or drawing) or photos of emotional expressions to match emotions on the wheel. Missing emotions can also be added with an associated emoji or expression. Machine research has found that facial expressions for sixteen major emotions are similar in all regions or cultures of the world.[10]
4. *Emotional Inquiry* is a deep and powerful process whereby students are invited to choose an emotion they have recently felt (or are feeling). They then inquire into what that feeling is trying to tell them and what could be learned from the feeling. See also *emotional gift research* (p. 198). Here are some examples of emotional inquiry:
   a. A feeling of subtle interest *helps make a choice* between two optional courses.
   b. A feeling of sadness on hearing a news story *clarifies a value or priority*.
   c. A feeling of wonder when hearing a guest speaker *reveals a desire* for a career.
   d. A feeling of irritation at a friend's flakiness *uncovers a need* for a boundary.

5. *Explore, compare, and connect* has pairs of students choose an emotion on the wheel, and find similar, opposite, or contrasting feelings. Qualities like intensity and duration can also be explored, as well as connections to songs, or stories that exemplify it. These findings can be shared back to the class orally or in written or visual form.
6. *Taste of Feeling* invites students to scan the feels wheel for an emotional experience they have had and are willing to resurface. The teacher may opt to focus on a particular group on the wheel: can you remember a time you felt any emotion within the anger section? As students recall the experience, invite them to sense what signals the body is sending and from where, taking on the expressions facially and in their bodies. Encourage a kind, accepting outlook toward these feelings and to any thoughts that arise with them.
7. *Emotional Journals* are periodic entries where feelings are recorded, along with the event(s) that caused them (or were triggered by them) as well as any insights, to develop emotional awareness and perspective. Feels wheels can help students find the right words for these journal entries.
8. *Labeling* uses the wheels to help put a specific word to feelings in the moment. This can happen any time in class before, during, or after learning. Labeling builds emotional vocabulary, provides insight into experiences, and reduces the emotional hijack felt with strong feelings. (Also see labeling with self-directed neuroplasticity, p. 156).
9. *Safety*: Students may have an unpleasant memory come up from simply seeing a particular emotion word or talking about it. Offer support, start slowly, and watch for those who indicate that they may need extra support.
10. *Integration Strategy*: Use feels wheels to help students talk about their feelings related to any learning task, curricular topic, assessment method, or teaching approach. This

includes all the remaining activities in this chapter, and other domains. Whether taking historical perspectives emotionally, or discerning feelings about any side of a curricular issue, consider the feels wheel an essential tool for regular school.

11. *Lifeplay*: Invite students to post the wheel at home and see what kind of conversation or openings it may create for emotional sharing.

Keywords: emotional, empower, identity, journal, foundational, integration, lifeplay, short-'n'-safe

Emotional Regulation(s)

"Never apologize for showing feelings. When you do so, you apologize for the truth."

—Benjamin Disraeli

There are no wrong emotions. Every feeling is the right one for us, in that moment. If a fear springs up, it might be a helpful warning to move to safety, or an echo of a past event wanting healing, or the very natural distress of being outside of one's comfort zone. Feelings may be surprising, unwanted, inconvenient, or all three. But they are always true.

That doesn't mean we don't have choices about how we flow with our feelings. One such choice is to *regulate* challenging emotional experiences by influencing the experience in some way, for ourselves or others (also see response-ability p. 123). Grade 7–12 students in particular can benefit from learning about this skill, as they encounter peaks and valleys of emotion through maturity. Regulation can be like filling the valleys with the peaks: going for a walk to calm down, or soothing a baby with a funny face. Listening and responding to emotional signals gives us a chance to adapt well, providing well-being benefits in a number of domains.[11]

Our emotional experience can feel more (or less) in harmony with the situation or surroundings we find ourselves in. For example, it's more socially acceptable to be playful at a park than at a funeral. While these unwritten rules can be broken, emotional regulation helps align with social regulations. Even making a choice to manage our feelings or not is a win in itself—a triumph of response-ability (see p. 115). This activity invites us to do what author Robert Kiyosaki suggests: "learn to use your emotions to think, not think with your emotions."

Summary: Discuss emotional regulation and its context and strategies in a community circle.
Time: 10–20 minutes
Trust Required: Low

1. *Circle Discussion* (10–20 minutes): Use some or all of the prompts below to explore emotional regulation(s), with students responding non-sequentially. Feels wheels are vital aids in helping students scan for feelings in response to the prompts. Consider opening the circle with a story of a time when you regulated an emotion. This could be in a professional or personal context, whichever feels best. Just as there are no wrong emotions, there are also no wrong answers to these questions.
    a. Read either of the quotations in this activity and ask if anyone can share a time when an emotion got the better of them.
    b. When or where might a particular emotion be more, or less, acceptable? Are there rules and regulations about emotions? If so, where do they come from?
    c. When is it helpful to regulate an emotion (which means to either influence, change, strengthen, or reduce it)? Give some examples such as calming down to avoid smashing something, dampening celebration when you've aced a test that your friend failed, or regulating between boredom and anxiety when studying.

>   d. Does anyone have any strategies for emotional regulation? Share some of your ideas and give a name to the strategy.
>   e. With regulation, it's possible to stop unhelpful reactions and even choose or change our response. Can anyone share an experience of doing this?
> 2. *Lifeplay*: Invite students to watch for emotional regulation in their lives, in themselves or others, as well as emotional regulations (spoken or unspoken). Debrief in class. See *response-ability* (p. 115) for much more on this.
>
> **Keywords**: circle, collaborative, emotional, lifeplay, prep-free, resilience, restorative, social, short-'n'-safe

E-motions: A Scavenger Hunt while Navigating the Road Trips and Roller Coasters of Life

> "Sunshine is delicious, rain is refreshing, wind braces us up, snow is exhilarating; there is really no such thing as bad weather, only different kinds of good weather."
>
> —John Ruskin

Most students and teachers would agree there *are* such things as bad emotions, and different kinds of good ones too. Our propensity to label emotions as bad or good is eclipsed only by our resistance to feeling them. The proto lingual root of emotion is *meue* (to push away), which became *movere* (to move). It is telling that our enduring human tendency has been to push away feelings or to move anywhere but nearer to the heart of them. This is especially true of bad experiences, but the good ones can also be resisted. Our defenses against feeling are numerous: attacking, avoiding, binging, blaming, denying, distracting, eating, escaping, faking, gaming, judging, laughing, helping, numbing, overworking, suppressing, or using.

Long-term avoidance, suppression (or any other defense), ultimately just stores up the unfelt feelings as emotional baggage. These trapped emotions result in negative physical, emotional, and social outcomes.[12] Clinging to good feelings has a similar effect of stopping our healthy flow. The turnaround is to find the motion in emotion: letting feelings *move us*, and then *move through us*. Karla McLaren, MEd, social science researcher and empathy pioneer, describes the gifts that feelings offer, when we can make this turn:

> Emotions are necessary—even when they're uncomfortable or socially inappropriate—because they are a part of your psyche, a part of your neural network, a part of your socialization, and a part of your humanity. Emotions aren't the enemy, but they have come to be vilified. . . . The only problem is that we truly need our emotions. We can't live functional lives without them. Without our emotions, we can't make decisions; we can't decipher our dreams and visions; we can't set proper boundaries or behave skillfully in relationships; we can't identify our hopes or support the hopes of others; and we can't connect to, or even find, our dearest loves.[13]

Whether uncomfortable or yummy, feelings are trying to tell us something. And unlike thoughts and behaviors, our feelings are always true. So to travel in the direction of well-being we need to turn toward our hearts and *feel*. This activity gives students and teachers a range of ways to be moved by, navigate, and befriend emotional experience. Whether a road trip or roller coaster, sharing aspects of our emotional life with a supportive group has much to offer: opening the door to well-being in many domains and helping us flow with the dance of emotion.[14]

Joy can be delicious, confusion can be refreshing, anger can brace us up, and fear can be exhilarating; there are really no such things as bad emotions, only different kinds of good emotions.

> **Summary**: Look for and reflect on emotional events during an extended e-motion scavenger hunt.
> **Time**: 10 minutes (initial), 5 minutes x 5+ (ongoing)
> **Trust Required**: Medium (varies with emotional comfort)
>
> 1. *Prep* (5 minutes): There is truly no preparing for e-motion, as our natural, healthy function is to flow with feelings each moment. However, teachers may wish to customize the events (rows) of this scavenger hunt (handout 7.1). Choose which events feel healthiest to include—or include them all.

Ensure students are familiar with the events chosen, or do other activities first to build familiarity, or remove them. Offer fun prizes for finding the first event, all the events, or having the best share. Keep it fun and light.

2. *Explain* (5 minutes): Explain that the class will be going on an e-motion scavenger hunt over a period of months. The invitation is to look for, learn about, and debrief a wide variety of emotional experiences whether felt oneself or observed in others. These might be encountered in or out of class. Pass out the scavenger hunts (handout 7.1) and put on your seat belt.
3. *Lifeplay*: This activity is primarily about lifeplay (observing and recording emotional events), although emotional experiences may come up in class. Let students know they need not point out observations they see in others, just note them and report back to the class as they wish.
4. *Debrief* (5 minutes): Debriefs happen any time a student (or teacher) wants to share an event they have found. These are learning moments to get into what happened, as well as thoughts, feelings (of course), impact, meaning, and what could change. Encourage on-the-fly research to find the gifts of particular emotions (see p. 198).
5. *Safety*: This activity is safer for groups who have built some community trust over time. Sharing, as always, is optional: students (and teacher) decide which experiences they will record and share, and which they won't. It may be difficult to find some events, so reassure the class that the goal is not to find them all but to expand one's repertoire of emotional experience.

Keywords: cognitive choice, emotional, lifeplay, mindfulness, resilience, support

Handout 7.1. E-motion Scavenger Hunt

Name: _____

Check off e-motional events you encounter in yourself or others. Write a word for the feeling on the blank line in the "Event" column and add insights about the experience in the other columns. Feel free to repeat any event by adding more checks, writing the feeling each time, and/or writing on the back.

E-motional Event	What happened? What did you feel? What stood out?	How could such an event contribute to wellness?	How could such an event take away from wellness?
feeling in myself ____			
feeling in another ____			
emotional inquiry ____			
interoception ____			
accepting a feeling with zero resistance ____			
feeling, but not sharing with anyone ____			
expressing a feeling by talking ____			
expressing a feeling with the whole body ____			
letting go of a feeling totally ____			
suppressing ____			
avoiding ____			
judging ____			
clinging ____			
regulating ____			

Fishbowl Circles: Appreciationships

"Everything the Power of the World does is done in a circle."

—Heȟáka Sápa

As classrooms make a shift in focus from head to heart, assessment can also shift from abstract products to more personal conversations and observations. The latter two are typically the shorter sides of assessment's write, say, do triangle, but open a valid and powerful window to next level learning.[15] When teachers observe students actually doing authentic classroom tasks, and engaging in rich conversations, it unveils the learning process itself, with all its attendant social and emotional aspects.

The fishbowl circle (see figure 7.2) blends conversation and observation to cultivate deep learning and emotional well-being. In the fishbowl, an inner circle of participants actively solves a problem, engages in a group task, or has a conversation. This inside circle could be a pair, small group, half the class, or more. While they interact, the outer circle gazes into the fishbowl, noticing learning moments, group processes, and more. Outer circle members may temporarily switch to a participant

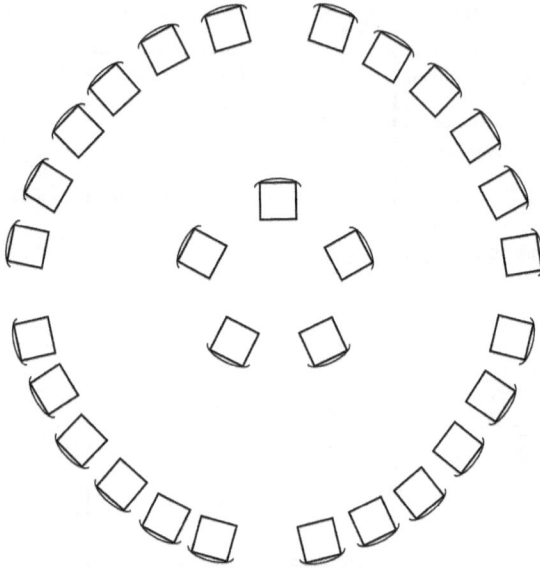

Figure 7.2. Fishbowl Circle

EMOTIONAL WELL-BEING

role by moving to an empty chair placed in the inner circle. Fishbowls can be used for a myriad of curriculum and well-being purposes.

This appreciationships activity described here is one such use, where the fishbowl is used to generate appreciation and elevation. The appreciationships activity works well with groups that have developed significant relationships over time, including staff. It is a profound gift to invite emotional expression in the appreciation of others, as the good feelings ripple out to all present. Activities that give future generations the courage to feel and share deeply, with the capacity to relate to emotions in themselves and others, could change everything. Indeed, transforming our emotional life could be what saves the world from ourselves.

> **Summary**: An inner circle conversing or doing something is observed by an outer circle.
> **Time**: 20+ minutes
> **Trust Required**: High
>
> 1. *Prep* (2 minutes): Create an inner circle of four to six chairs, plus an additional empty chair. Surround this group with an outer circle for the remainder of the class, which can often be a standing circle for simplicity.
> 2. *Explain roles* (1 minute): The inside group will respond to the prompts (see step 3), while the outside circle is asked to observe quietly, and make notes if desired, about the emotional cues and body language associated with different feelings (e.g., gratitude, joy, elevation). Outside circle participants can also temporarily take the empty seat in the inside circle if they wish to contribute, then return to their outer circle.
> 3. *Appreciationships* (12 minutes): The first person in the inside circle is asked, "What does being in this (class/group/team) mean to you?" and given a minute to respond. After this, the other members of the inner circle then take turns responding to "What do you appreciate about (first person)?" for about thirty seconds each. After everyone in the inside circle has appreciated the first person (a few minutes), the process is

repeated with each other person in the inside circle until everyone has been appreciated. Outside circle members may swap in to add their appreciations as well.
4. After this demonstration/fishbowl circle, the class can be split into groups to repeat the process so everyone, including the teacher, is involved. Those in the first group can act as single observers to each other circle.
5. *Debrief* (5 minutes): Use the standard debrief questions (p. 16) or the prompts below, being sure to solicit comments from the outside as well as inside circle:
    a. Do we often say what we really feel and think about others, even if it's kind?
    b. What is the impact of sharing appreciation on giver, receiver, and observers?
    c. Why do we share? Why do we hold back?
6. *Safety*: While appreciationships work best with high trust groups, fishbowl circles can be used in a variety of ways that don't require deep bonds (table 7.1). The teacher can also strategically choose which group to join in order to ensure a good experience for all.
7. *Integration Strategy*: Fishbowls are fantastic for a wide range of cross-curricular and schoolwide purposes, wherever observation, conversation, or deeper aspects of learning are involved (see table 7.1 for examples).
8. *Schoolwide Extension*: Staff meetings, town halls, or other events can use fishbowls to explicitly surface and explore emotional, social, and deeper processes.

Keywords: caring, cognitive, circle, collaborative, choice, emotional, gratitude, hedonia, integration, lifeplay, schoolwide, social, space, support

EMOTIONAL WELL-BEING

Table 7.1 Fishbowl Strategies

Type	Inner Circle	Outer Circle	Examples
Conversations	Discuss, debate, or have a dialogue to explore any topic in the curriculum (especially richer, nuanced, or abstract curricular aspects).	Observe and note higher order thinking (inference, analysis, metacognition, synthesis, evaluation), and emotional cues (verbal or nonverbal).	Media studies advertisement case, analyzing a political speech, discussing geographical factors on food production.
Observations	Small group works at a curricular task perhaps using chart paper or whiteboard.	Watches for social dynamics (questioning, affirming, adding on, paraphrasing) and/or higher-order skills (curricular processes like problem solving).	Create an impromptu drama piece, solve a science problem, discuss a business case, mock up coding (on a whiteboard).
Troubleshooting	One person shares a problem or dilemma they are facing, without being interrupted. Inner members respond to the problem, while the original person listens. Final word goes to the original person.	Watch for and describe clues that indicate confusion, empathy, kindness, optimism, trust, surprise, interest, or any other emotion. Swap into the inner circle to offer a perspective on the dilemma.	In a staff meeting, teachers could share a persistent classroom challenge or issue. In a classroom, students could describe aspects of learning (or life) they are struggling with in some way.

Heartwarming

Being kind to others is universally accepted as a virtuous act, and many people do it quite well. On the other hand, being kind to *oneself* has mixed reviews, and many people struggle to do it at all. Sharon Salzberg opens the door to this paradox when she wrote, "You could search the whole world over and never find anyone as deserving of your love as yourself." But to walk through that door, we need simple practices that nourish our very own bodies, minds, hearts, and souls—like *Heartwarming*.

> **Summary**: Generate warmth for different aspects of oneself with a series of affectionate touches.
> **Time**: 4 minutes
> **Trust Required**: Low
>
> 1. *Warm-up* (30 seconds): Invite the class to take a comfortable seat, perhaps dimming the lights, and use or adapt the following script. "Close your eyes if you wish, and gently rub your palms together, feeling some warmth building in your hands."
> 2. *Mind* (30 seconds): "Cup your cheeks lightly with your hands, and let some warmth spread. Send some gratitude and love to your marvelous, magnificent mind. A mind that can solve problems, create, imagine, and dream, and without which you wouldn't be alive, let alone enjoy life. Give some love and appreciation to your mind." After a short pause, ask students to re-warm their palms by gently rubbing again.
> 3. *Heart* (30 seconds): "Now cross your hands over your heart, and let some warmth spread. Send some gratitude and love to your marvelous, magnificent heart. A heart that keeps your life blood flowing and can feel all the experiences of life sensitively and deeply. Generate some love and appreciation for your heart." After a short pause, ask students to re-warm their palms by gently rubbing again.

4. *Body* (30 seconds): "Now put your hands on your belly, and let some warmth spread. Send some gratitude and love to your marvelous, magnificent body. A body that is your vehicle in this life, through which you sense and interact with the world in so many ways. Generate some love and appreciation for your body." After a short pause, ask students to re-warm their palms by gently rubbing again.
5. *Self* (30 seconds): "Now wrap your arms around yourself and give yourself a big hug, and let some warmth spread. Send some gratitude and love to your entire, marvelous, magnificent self: mind, heart, body, and soul. Hold this feeling for a little while and feel all your aspects warming."
6. *Debrief* (1–2 minutes): Use the questions to debrief anything (p. 16) and then ask if any particular aspect (mind, heart, body, self/soul) felt easier or more resistant.
7. *Lifeplay*: At any time when you're sitting or just waiting somewhere, cup your cheek or take any of the other postures to let some silent warmth and love flow.

Keywords: card, caring, cognitive, emotional, gratitude, hedonia, lifeplay mindfulness, prep-free, restorative, short-n'-safe

Taking Back "How Are You?"

How are you? How's it going? How're you doing?! These questions are so commonplace that a reply isn't even expected, and when one comes, it is usually trivial rather than genuine. This activity takes back these questions by transforming them from superficial greetings into openings for emotional intimacy. If these phrases are used as they are literally intended, an opportunity to connect deeply arises. Sharing deeper thoughts and feelings nourishes emotional well-being and provides a choice: exchange a simple greeting or share how we truly are.

Summary: Pair up and take turns responding to "How are you?" in different ways.
Time: 10 minutes
Trust Required: High

1. *Everyday Greeting Version* (1 minute): Pair up students, have them face each other, and use or adapt the following script: "I'm going to ask a question and I invite everyone to respond to their partner naturally and immediately, without thinking. Both partners can reply at the same time. Ready? Ok, here's the question [dramatic pause] . . . How are you?" Typical responses might be "fine," "okay," or "good," or "how are you?"
2. *Intimate Version* (5 minutes): "Now you will ask each other the same question 'How are you?,' but this time taking two minutes for each person to respond deeply and authentically as they wish. Each partner gets a turn speaking (while the other listens) for two minutes. The person sitting closest to the door will ask the question first, and then I'll prompt you to switch." Use a timer to ensure each person gets their turn. The two minutes may be extended for deeper sharing, although it can feel like a long time for some people.
3. *Debrief* (5 minutes): Invite partners to debrief as a pair first, then with the whole group.
   a. *What happened? Thoughts? Feelings?* Contrast the superficial/greeting version with the intimate version of the experience.
   b. *What is our purpose in asking these questions?* If we wish to greet someone, saying "nice to see you" or some other greeting may be more appropriate. At other times, we may genuinely want to connect more deeply and ask a question.
   c. *How do we typically answer these kinds of questions?* How does it feel to share deeply? Are we encouraged to do so on a regular basis?

4. *Safety*: Sharing emotional states authentically requires significant vulnerability (for the sharer) and sensitivity (for the listener). Emphasize that depth (or shallowness) of sharing is always according to each person's comfort and safety.
5. *Lifeplay*: Challenge the entire class (students and teacher alike) to consider responding deeply when they hear these phrases, and also consider their intention on using them. Debrief this challenge to see what happens when we consider carefully whether to simply greet, or deeply inquire, when we meet another person.

Keywords: caring, emotional, icebreaker, lifeplay, prep-free, support

SUPPLEMENTARIES: SHORT, SIMPLE, SAFE, OR SEARCHABLE EMOTIONAL WELL-BEING

- *The Atlas of Emotions* provides a beautiful visual of the emotional world, complete with simple examples of how prior experience, context, triggering events, emotions, and awareness all contribute toward our capacity to respond.[16] While not quite a feels wheel, the atlas can serve a different purpose by illustrating the mechanism and modifiers of emotional response. *Search terms*: atlas emotions.
- *Circle Games* are sources of joy and emotional learning wrapped up in the fun and familiar context of game playing. Debriefing what happened after the game (optional) can help get deeper with emotional experience. Pause the game and start a discussion when a magical teaching/learning moment (MTLM) arises (see p. 14). With so many games to explore (see search terms), there are many opportunities to talk about feelings or just play a game. The games listed are relatively low risk, but others may require higher trust, especially those requiring physical touch, such as the human knot. See also circle energizers (p. 229) for lighter and simpler warmups. *Search terms*: circle, games, youth.

- *Crossed/Uncrossed* passes a pair of sticks around a circle, with the facilitator asking each person to hold them and say out loud "crossed" or "uncrossed." Here's the secret: however the sticks are held, and whatever the person says, the facilitator will confirm "yes, crossed" only if the *legs* of the person are crossed, otherwise saying "nope, uncrossed." As the sticks circulate, feelings of confusion, determination, frustration, anger, curiosity, and elation may arise. The debrief could explore these feelings, along with the need to be in the know and our willingness (or unwillingness) to experience *not knowing*. Groups of teachers can especially benefit from this game, providing an experience of not knowing.
- *I Like My Neighbor* starts with the teacher removing their chair from the circle, stepping into the middle and calling out "I like my neighbor who is jeans" or "I like my neighbor who has short hair" or "I like my neighbor who is wearing red." All those matching the statement jump up to find another chair, and whomever is left chairless must make the next "I like my neighbor" statement. Debrief around feelings of being in the middle—or avoiding it at all costs—and how we are the same or different.
- *Going on a Picnic* is similar to crossed/uncrossed, but with a different secret. Students in the circle are told there is going to be a picnic and then asked sequentially what they may bring. The facilitator responds to what is being brought by saying "yes, you may come" (if their item begins with the same letter as their first name) or "sorry, you may not come" (otherwise). For example if Emma says she's bringing eggs, she may come. If Noah also tries to bring eggs, he's not invited. Debrief feelings of inclusion, exclusion, being in the know (or not), and whatever else arises emotionally.

- *Emotional Gift Research* recognizes that every feeling has something to offer. Even the most devastating experiences can result in growth, clarify values, or push a person to healthy transformation. For example, sadness is a key emotion for letting go of what we are holding onto, so we can open up again. Grief also clarifies what is meaningful to us, as we recognize and celebrate what was lost. Shame can show us where we have violated our personal boundaries and values. Using feels wheels, have students do some quick research and report back to the class, or search on-the-fly when

an emotion comes up in class to learn more about its gifts. *Search terms*: [emotion], value, importance, gifts, teach.
- *Emotional Well-Being Apps* track moods, inspire gratitude, help practice self-help skills, and more. For classroom use, try free apps designed for young people that protect privacy and promote positive, research-based approaches. Otherwise, let students use their own in consultation with caregivers or mental health professionals. *Search terms*: teenage, youth, app, [mood, gratitude, feelings, emotion]
- *Feelings Maps* let students work in small groups to brainstorm and/or research emotional indicators, and write them on a simple outline of the human body. For example, orange can be used for joy, drawing arrows to a smiling mouth, flushed face, or other signs of joy all in orange. The teacher can divide up feelings by group, or let the entire class work on a single, mural paper on the floor, using a human-sized outline (the teacher can be the model). See also "Stress Signals," p. 140.
- *Give a Little Bit* of your life by sharing an appropriate personal story now and then, including the emotional components, to encourage students to do the same. For example, how did you become a teacher, and why do you love (or not) your subject?
- *Gratitudinals* are simple expressions of the all-star practice and emotion of gratitude. Gratitude boosts well-being in the joy of noticing and appreciating what's good in this world, but also by adding to life satisfaction, better sleep, quality relationships, and reduced stress.[17] Gratitude practices were as effective as clinical interventions to reduce anxiety or improve body image, as well as more likely to be actually practiced.
  - *Gratitude Lists* are a classic practice of students (and the teacher) writing a few things to be grateful for each day. This can be done in a diary, device, or journal at whatever time works best. Brainstorming a few ideas as a class can kickstart the practice.
  - *Gratitude Murals* on the classroom wall or even in the school halls can be left open for anyone to add sticky notes or expressions of appreciation.
  - *Appreciation Contemplation* is to pause and notice something good for a minute or so, often leading to a mental sequence of grateful thoughts. When practiced as many times a day as feels

helpful, a positive (rather than lack-oriented) mindset is induced that persists and grows over time.
- ○ *Acts of Gratitude* could be verbal thank-yous, hand-delivered letters, or any other act of appreciation that shows someone how much they matter. The resulting elevation (see p. 66) can also inspire more of the same.
- ○ *Thank, Not Bank* is to refrain from acquiring something new, instead appreciating what one already has. Fewer material things may reduce stress for some.
- *Joy Jars* hold slips of paper with happy moments from class, jokes, or positive sayings written on them. These can be read out any time someone needs some joy or toward the end of the year. Variations could be the "Grateful Jar" or "Compliments Jar."
- *Love Song to Self* is a surprising practice, both for its incredible impact but also in its uniqueness, since most love songs are not self-reflective. Get students to choose favorite love songs and play a medley of them in class (maybe 30 seconds of each one), inviting them to close their eyes and imagine they are *singing the words to themselves*. A debrief isn't necessary to know the impact of imagining the song is both *for* you and *from* you.
- *Name It to Tame It* is an emotional regulation process from Dr. Dan Siegel that involves naming emotions verbally, especially when they are felt strongly. Like labeling (see p. 154), identifying an emotion by naming it can help avoid getting caught up in the feeling, and remain a little calmer.
- *Pretending to Be Funny* recognizes that comedic skills are not the signature strength of every teacher, but YouTube can be a great substitute. Show a video, project a cartoon, tell stories, find a meme, make fun of yourself (never students), and create a lightness that carries through their lives. Students can take turns choosing material, with teacher moderation. For next-level comedy, use classroom moments as opportunities to develop improvisational humor chops. *Search terms*: improv, rules, basics, beginner.
- *Self-Compassion Practices* rank right up there with gratitude as a fabulous practice of well-being. Self-compassion provides benefits galore in the emotional, physical, cognitive, resilience, and social domains.[18] By blending emotional awareness (p. 182) with the equanimity to kindly hold oneself (p. 194), self-compassion uses

kindness as a response to personal suffering or perceived flaws. Self-compassion can be gentle and caring or firmer and bolstering, whatever feels best. The key is to see that we all suffer, such that the distinction between self-compassion and compassion (self and other) blurs. Here are some simple ways students and teachers can develop self-compassion:

- *Affirmations* may feel good for some. Invite students to find one they like and set it as the wallpaper of their phone. *Search terms*: positive affirmations self
- *Comforting Oneself* physically or mentally is self-compassionate. Try self-massage (p. 231), mindfulness moments (p. 145), heart-warming (p. 194), or look through the entire self-care index (p. 293).
- *Love Text to Self* is a loving text message sent to self, including whatever feels painful but also what's great about yourself, and why you love yourself. Invite the class to write the text in first or third person, whichever feels more loving, send it, and then have them scroll back and re-read the text throughout the term.
- *Friend to Self* is to think of what you would say to a good friend whom you cared about if they were in your situation, then direct these compassionate words to oneself, either verbally or as a written reflection.

- *Words of Feeling* invites students to practice kind awareness while listening to feeling words spoken aloud. Start with milder feelings, and give students an out to just put in earbuds and meditate silently if they wish. Use this script, then debrief:
  - "Close your eyes and get comfortable. I will say a series of words for different feelings. As you hear each one, just notice what happens, if anything. Focus on the body without putting any effort into thinking. Imagine you are a boat with a deep keel of awareness, if a word hits you like a big wave, you may get rocked a bit, but your keel keeps you steady."
  - Speak some of the words leaving 10–20 seconds in between each one.
  - "Happy, sad, joyful, frightened, excited, anxious, peaceful, bored, restless, eager, doubtful, strong, weak, curious, serious, worried, lonely, envious, mischievous, disappointed, angry, hateful, grateful, loving."

8

ENVIRONMENTAL WELL-BEING

Wellness with the Natural World

> "Action on behalf of life transforms. Because the relationship between self and the world is reciprocal, it is not a question of first getting enlightened or saved and then acting. As we work to heal the earth, the earth heals us."[1]
>
> —Joanna Macy

The coronavirus pandemic forced education to change its seating plan en masse, moving learning online all over the world. But the pandemic also pushed classes outdoors, just as with the 19th-century tuberculosis epidemic. These moves kept schools running and reduced illness. While learning online increases computer time, outdoor learning addresses this second epidemic that impacts children and youth: excessive screen time.[2] Outdoor learning reveals what our bodies already know: that wellness in multiple domains is related to closeness with the natural world, of which we are an inseparable part.[3]

Outdoor learning isn't just week-long canoe trips or outdoor adventure experiences such as ropes courses, it includes any educational experience that happens outside. At school, this could look like reading time under the trees in the yard or an outdoor classroom lesson. Beyond the school, a walk on a nature path, a field trip to the wetlands, or a full credit in outdoor education can all help make the shift from screen to green. Cultivating environmental well-being is about so much more than just being "outdoorsy."

Our personal sense of connection with nature, concern for the environment, and affinity for spending time outdoors collectively make up our *nature relatedness* (NR). These qualities are correlated to a number of well-being domains, as those with higher degrees of NR tend to

- be more social, trusting, helpful, conscientious, and open-minded;[4]
- have higher awareness, self-acceptance, emotional well-being, and social well-being;[5]
- feel eudaimonic well-being in terms of autonomy, purpose, and personal growth;[6]
- have more physical and cognitive energy;[7] and
- see connection with nature as a transcendent, spiritual experience.

These benefits link to seven other domains of well-being, making environmental wellness an exceptionally integrated realm of student thriving. This individual flourishing extends to the Earth itself, as those with strong NR protect the environment, take action to live sustainably, and help others do the same. Learning outdoors cultivates a caring stewardship for the natural world that is our home, while also fostering personal wellness. More powerfully, nature connectedness is a key correlate to transcendent experiences, providing a doorway to the spiritual domain.[8]

Elizabeth Nisbet, environmental and health researcher, conveys the breadth of this dynamic between humans and the natural world:

> Nature relatedness is an appreciation for and understanding of our interconnectedness with all other living things on Earth. NR is distinct from environmentalism in that it is comprised of much more than activism. Nor is it simply a love for nature, or enjoyment of only the superficially pleasing facets of nature, such as sunsets and snowflakes. NR is an understanding of the importance of all aspects of nature, even those that are not aesthetically appealing or useful to humans, such as mosquitoes, mice, death, and decay.[9]

The United Kingdom took this to heart in 2012 by embracing learning outdoors, opening forest/nature schools, and creating outdoor learning

ENVIRONMENTAL WELL-BEING

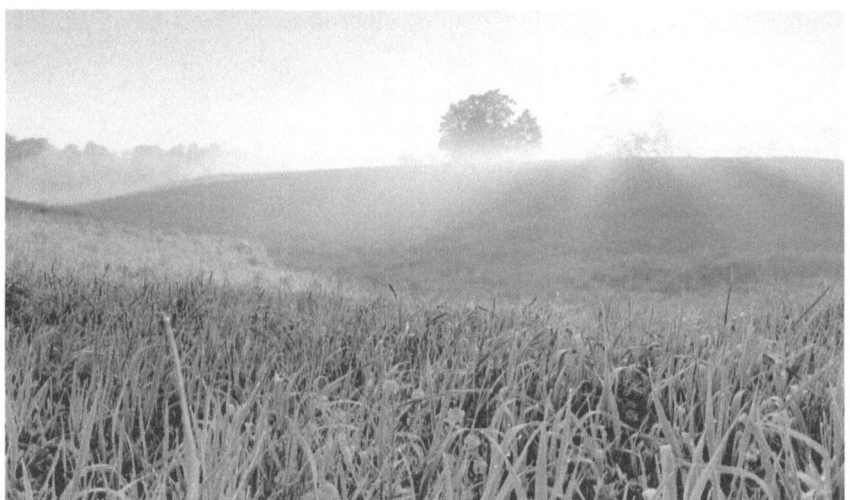

Figure 8.1. Nature relatedness connects to every domain of well-being.

spaces. These innovations overcame some long-held and undeserved stigmas that outdoor learning is inherently risky and costly.[10]

After four years of demonstration projects, 92 percent of teachers said students were more engaged with outdoor learning, 85 percent saw an improvement in behavior, and 90 percent of students reported feeling happier and healthier when learning outdoors.[11] Nigeria, Germany, Canada, and most Nordic countries have followed the United Kingdom in developing widespread outdoor learning programs.[12]

Environmental well-being efforts can also be aided by abundant resources and partners beyond the school. These include outdoor education programs, parks at all levels of government, and non-governmental organizations such as the Nature Conservancy. District consultants may support environmental education directly or facilitate connections to local experts including Indigenous knowledge keepers. Ancestral knowledge can help build student understanding and respect for Indigenous peoples, perspectives, and the natural world we all share.

As learning is shifted outdoors, students can begin to appreciate our precious, vulnerable, and ultimate sources of wellness: air, water, plants, and animals. As nature appreciation matures, so too does the desire to protect it. As nature education author David Sobel writes, "If we want children to flourish, to become truly empowered, then let us allow them to love the earth before we ask them to save it." Personal and natural wellness cannot be separated, making environmental well-being a priority for all classrooms on planet Earth.

Key Messages

- Environmental well-being isn't just outdoor education (as a program), but any education that happens outdoors, including on school grounds and in the natural world beyond.
- Nature relatedness (NR) consists of a person's understanding of nature, feelings of love for nature, and affinity for being in, and protecting, the natural world.
- NR correlates to well-being in numerous domains, including the physical, cognitive, emotional, eudaimonic, resilience, social, and spiritual.
- Environmental well-being through learning outdoors can be safe, affordable, and supported by resources in the district and community.

ENVIRONMENTAL WELL-BEING ACTIVITIES

Walk the Talk (Main Move)

> "Symphony starts when you walk together, feel the heartbeats, and understand the unspoken words."
>
> —Amit Ray

Being outside changes the energy of group interactions. Just sitting outdoors in nature with space stretching in all directions adds qualities unavailable in a closed classroom. In walking, people move in one direction together rather than fixed in opposition at a table. Power dynamics shift with movement, and walking outdoors boosting multiple elements of physical, emotional, cognitive, and social well-being.[13] Outdoor walking meetings in particular heighten creativity, increase energy, and improve communication.[14]

Students and staff receptiveness to scheduling a meeting on a walk, or taking a class outside for group discussions, increases by doing it, and realizing benefits. Whether strolling the school grounds, lapping the

ENVIRONMENTAL WELL-BEING

track, or following a path through a natural area, walking the talk invites a whole new perspective, building environmental and group connections in the process.

> **Summary**: Hold small meetings, group work, and one-on-one partner tasks outside while walking.
> **Time**: Varies
> **Trust Required**: Low
>
> 1. *Pre-Class Prep*: Choose a route near green spaces, quieter areas, and where people can walk side-by-side as possible, considering accessibility needs. Online mapping tools can estimate the time needed for a route, but even repeated laps around the school track are beneficial. Add routes with their length and duration to the school room booking system to promote getting outside.
> 2. *Integration Strategy*: Outside walks can integrate with many classroom activities, particularly small group work if not whole-class lessons. Groups of two or three are the sweet spot, although slightly larger groups can work if there is space to walk abreast and/or the surroundings are relatively quiet. Partner discussions, micro labs (p. 129) or group brainstorming work well, especially with more space to spread out and eliminate the noise level that would be produced in a typical classroom setting.
> 3. *In-Class Prep* (1 minute): Explain that the next activity will be outside and whether to leave bags or phones in the locked classroom. Tell students they must remain in sight of the teacher, have a signal to regroup, and bring what materials they need (usually phones can access materials or take notes). Give the activity instructions, such as "pick up a playing card on the way out, find your group of three by card rank, then brainstorm all the ways you use electricity at school or at home. This recorder is whomever got the hearts card on their card recording for the group." As students get accustomed to walking the talk, setup quickens.

4. *Outside* (varies): Monitor groups to ensure they stay in view and on task. Use the signal to gather students for instructions, consolidate learning, or debrief. Break up longer periods of small-group walking in this way or go back to the classroom.
5. *Safety and Accessibility*: Ensure everyone can participate well, planning a break if there is a route. Let groups know ahead of time, so they can plan footwear, dress, or bring a water bottle. Keep routes within school grounds for student walks, or do the paperwork to permit informal walks around the school neighborhood, if that is desirable. Manage strong sun with hats, shade from trees or shelters, and avoid the hottest part of the day.
6. *Schoolwide Extension*: Use walking meetings with staff committees, school clubs, or any group that normally sits around a table and talks. Meetings of two to five can happen well on a walk outside, especially where mobile devices suffice for meeting needs. This also applies to virtual meetings, where participants can be outdoors and still participate.

Keywords: card, cognitive, collaborative, emotional, environmental, foundational, hedonia, integration, outdoor, physical, schoolwide, social, space

Nature Immersion

"To observe without evaluating is the highest form of intelligence."

—Jiddu Krishnamurti

The tendency to label, describe, and classify can get in the way of directly experiencing the natural world. Our capacity to purely sense an experience can be lost in the chatter of mental commentary about it. In this activity, students get quiet, up close, and personal with nature to cultivate awareness and peacefulness, and discover what is not always describable in words.

Summary: Mindfully experience an aspect of nature.
Time: 15 minutes
Trust Required: Low

1. *Prep*: Teachers choose an element of nature near the school for a mindful immersion. This could be a tree with branches close to the ground, a patch of uncut grass or meadow with a variety of plants, a place where birds gather, or just a moss-covered rock.
2. *Mindfulness* (5 minutes): After taking students to the chosen site, begin with some grounding or centering practices, using any one of the mindfulness moments (see p. 145) to help students access their awareness. Invite sensing without thinking or labeling, just taking everything in without mental or spoken dialogue. Conduct a lengthier 5-4-3-2-1 guided experience with the natural element (see p. 155). For example, standing in the boughs of a white pine, what are five things you can see, four things you can hear, three things you can touch, two smells, and one feeling inside your body?
3. *Focus Elements* (5 minutes): Invite students to choose a particular sense to focus on, such as having them close their eyes and *feel* the natural element without any talking. In the case of the white pine, they may roll the needles in their fingers and notice the triangular shape, count the needles per bundle, or immerse themselves in the texture of the bark. Repeat this step for other senses as desired or let students freely sense. Maintain silence, and encourage a kind awareness, without any intention of thinking.
4. *Debrief* (5 minutes): Have students self-reflect, journal, and/or share what they learned or what came up for them in the immersion. Reflections may be about nature (such as the impact of the season on the immersion) or the nature of being with something mindfully.
5. *Safety*: Our ancestors relied on foraging for food before modern agriculture and food distribution, making foraging a

wonderful way to reconnect with nature. However, students should not eat anything, even if it is edible. Taste can be sensed through scent, such as by rubbing pine needles between the fingers near the nose.
6. *Integration Strategy*: Consider connections between the natural element and your curriculum. For example, a Fermi problem involving the number of needles in a pine forest or measuring the height of the tree indirectly with trigonometry.
7. *Lifeplay*: Invite students to use their encounters with the natural world, however brief, as cues to take in experience purely, without the need to label, name, or think about it. Just seeing the sky walking home from school, a bird streak silently through the sky, or hearing rainfall can become transformative experiences of peace and beauty when the mind stills.

Keywords: choice, environmental, integration, journal, lifeplay, mindfulness, outdoor, space, spiritual

SUPPLEMENTARIES: SHORT, SIMPLE, SAFE, OR SEARCHABLE ENVIRONMENTAL WELL-BEING

"Time in nature is not leisure time; it's an essential investment in our children's health."[15]

—Richard Louv

- *SMARTER Eco-Action* applies the SMARTER goal process (p. 100) to an environmental effort in the classroom or school (see eco clubs below). Students can work in small groups by interest, pursuing a project or goal that sustains nature, using resources efficiently, promoting learning and activism, or preventing harm to the environment.
- *Bring Nature In* recognizes that schools without outdoor classrooms, or with very limited access to natural spaces, can bring a piece of the natural world inside. Open window views, plants, terrariums, stone gardens, or other natural features can sooth and

beautify the classroom.[16] Nature photos or a projected nature scene (forest, mountain, meadow, or ocean) are better than nothing. See "A Loving Container" (p. 47) for more ideas.
- *Earth/Eco/Green/Environment Clubs* empower committed students and teachers to create environmental wellness for the school community and the earth. Through action planning, schoolwide initiatives, and educational efforts, such clubs can create green spaces, reduce waste or energy use, and support outdoor learning. Widespread support and resources for such groups is available from educational and environmental organizations. Even the United Nations support such clubs as part of their sustainable development goals.[17] *Search terms*: environment, club, school.
- *Forest Schools* are outdoor education programs that visit woodlands or natural settings. Forest JK-SK programs were a natural first, with kindergarten literally meaning "children garden." Typically students engage in cross-curricular learning, holistic personal development, and social-emotional well-being. *Search term:* forest school.
- *Going Green (Give One, Get One)* uses a sheet of recycled paper folded in half to make a "give one" side and a "get one" side. Individually, students are asked to write down ideas regarding some aspect of greening on the "give one" side (e.g., how to connect with nature, save energy, reduce waste, etc.). They then circulate, finding partners (or small groups) to share one of their ideas with and receiving new ideas from others. These are recorded on the "get one" side along with the name of the giver. Follow up in a week's time to provide accountability to implementing one or more of the ideas.
- *Outdoor Classrooms* can be a schoolwide venture or a single-class project that boosts outdoor learning and gives students places to be with their friends outside of class. More involved efforts involve tree planting, accompanying gardens, an amphitheater, or armor stone seating. A simple option is providing log slice seating for flexible groups and circles, placed and spaced for optimal hearing. Collaborate with administrators, teachers, students, parents, and community partners to plan and seek funding. *Search terms:* outdoor classroom.

- *Outside the Box* takes individual work time (including silent reading, writing assignments, math seat work, and more) outside. Students bring whatever materials, books and writing tools they need, including personal phones or school devices if necessary. Spreading out on the grass, lying against trees, or sitting on some rocks to get some work done can bring a revitalizing change to typical seatwork "in the box."
- *Rewilding* transforms a typical fenced-in, grass-and-asphalt schoolyard by adding native plants, gardens, large logs to sit and play on, trees for blossoms and shade, or even allowing access to woodland areas where possible. If a classroom has a door to the outside, consider adding a small garden just outside that door to create a space for students to learn, rest, or play. Rewilding helps rebalance school priorities of maintenance, surveillance, and risk aversion to include natural wellness.
- *Walk and Roll* encourages walking or biking to school for both students and staff. Increasing pedestrian and bike traffic curbs vehicular congestion, reduces pollution, and increases wellness in a number of domains (see "Walk the Talk," p. 206). Funding may be available from municipal programs, government grants, or a charity week (collect donations from those who use the parking lot). When more people walk and roll together, the environmental and physical wellness is complemented with social well-being and community connection. These efforts can be simple, or more widespread, potentially involving the whole school and community:
    - arranging a walk/bike week or buddy program where people travel in groups;
    - run programs that provide and/or repair student bicycles and teach cycling safety;
    - install bike racks or additional walking paths near the school;
    - start a "walking bus" or bicycle convoy program; or
    - provide education about the benefits of not driving, with or without contests.

    Search terms: bike, walk to school, programs.

9

PHYSICAL WELL-BEING

Healthy Bodies, Balanced Lifestyles

> "Health is a state of complete physical, mental and social well-being and not merely the absence of disease or infirmity."[1]
>
> —World Health Organization

Good health was traditionally all about exercise and nutrition. And yet as more love goes to cognitive, emotional, and social well-being, it only becomes clearer that every domain supports physical wellness, and vice versa. Physical health weaves with every aspect of thriving, and yet grade 7–12 students have increasingly unhealthy bodies and body images. Some focus on the body to the point of disorder; others neglect multiple aspects of physical health:

- 80 percent of young people aged 11–17 get insufficient daily physical activity;[2]
- 60 percent of middle schoolers, and 70 percent of high schoolers don't get enough sleep, and this trend has been worsening;[3]
- 67 percent of adolescents had a poor diet in 2016;[4] and
- 80 percent of 17-year-old girls are unhappy with their body.[5]

Adult statistics are better, but the bodies of educators and students in general could benefit from more movement, longer rest, and good fuel—the major pillars of physical well-being. If you are lucky enough to be a physical education, health, or family studies teacher, you have a great deal of influence in these areas. Acknowledging this good work, the activities in this shorter chapter give other classroom teachers some opportunities to support a well-known, if sometimes neglected, pillar of wellness that is so central to flourishing.

Key Messages

- Youth and adolescent health is in serious decline, with significant and widespread issues in every pillar of physical well-being: movement/exercise, diet/nutrition, and sleep/rest.
- Physical well-being supports most every other domain of well-being, and vice versa.

PHYSICAL WELL-BEING ACTIVITIES

Puzzling Out Wellness with Jigsaw Accountability Groups (Main Move)

> "The American mind in particular has been trained to equate success with victory, to equate doing well with beating someone. . . . It is possible to achieve mastery of a problem or a skill without hurting another person or even without attempting to conquer."
>
> —Elliot Aronson

Segregation in American schools didn't end with the 1954 Supreme Court decision *Brown v. Board of Education of Topeka*. In many places, like Austin, Texas, it was only the beginning of decades of resistance to integration. In 1971, federal government lawsuits forced the district's hand, so they closed schools with only black students and bussed them across the city to all-white schools. This one-way policy didn't end the struggle for racial and educational equity, but it's where psychologist Elliot Aronson got involved—by being given a puzzle.

PHYSICAL WELL-BEING

With racial violence flaring in the newly integrated schools, the superintendent reached out in desperation to his former professor, Aronson, for help. Classrooms at the time, integrated or not, had little or no cooperation or interaction between students. There were also deep-seated racial biases. Aronson's solution to this puzzle was to create his own puzzle: the jigsaw classroom. For two months, students were put in mixed, cooperative groups. The results were increased empathy across racial lines, higher morale, and better attendance. Students in minority groups also had significant academic improvement, especially those in lower income families.[6]

This activity uses the prosocial structure of Aronson's jigsaw innovation to explore aspects of physical health while building social capital. It also lays down another important piece: student choice in a cooperative task that improves, not just teaches, physical wellness.

> **Summary**: Use jigsaw accountability to learn about, and improve, physical well-being.
> **Time**: 5–10 minutes x 4–7 classes over a period of weeks
> **Trust Required**: Medium
>
> 1. *Prep* (5 minutes): Select six or more online quizzes or surveys on the pillars of physical health for youth (see pillar quizzes for details p. 231). Quiz topics could be breaks and rest, cardio, eating disorders, flexibility, hygiene, leisure and structured exercise, macronutrients, medical care, sexual health, sleep, strength training, substance (ab)use, water intake, and more. If desired, focus on one pillar by finding quizzes only about diet and nutrition. Make the quiz links available electronically for students or print copies.
> 2. *Brief* (5 minutes): Ask students to write down the pillars of physical well-being individually. After a moment, invite some responses, then share that the major pillars are movement/exercise, food for fuel and enjoyment, and sleep. Like with many subjects, teens will have a wide range of understanding (or not) in these pillars.

3. *Quiz* (5 minutes): Students choose one of the quizzes from step 1 above to complete personally, as does the teacher. When the quizzes are completed, debrief any insights, new learning, or debunked myths from the quiz results. Tally privately how many chose each quiz (see p. 40) to find the top interests. Tell students that over the next few weeks they will be going on a physical wellness J.A.G. (jigsaw accountability group) that will involve the following:
   a. depending on each other to learn about the topics (jigsaw); and
   b. supporting each other in personal goals related to the topics (accountability).
4. *Jigsaw Home Groups* (5 minutes): Divide students into visibly random (p. 84) home groups with the size of each group being the number of quiz topics chosen. Join one of the groups as a teacher if that is helpful. Each group member picks one of the topics so they are all covered (rock, paper, scissors can break disagreements).
5. *Jigsaw Expert Groups* (10 minutes): Reform the class into expert groups by topic. Expert groups then research their topic, citing reliable sources. Groups know they are done when they come up with the following:
   a. *Three very important points (V.I.P.s)* about their topic. For example, on hydration, one point could be that optimal hydration is gauged by light (nearly clear) urine.
   b. *Three quiz questions*, with answers, students can use to check understanding. For example, "What percentage of daily water do we get from food?" (Answer: 20 percent)
   c. *Three personal actions* (one simple, one moderate, and one involved) to improve well-being in that topic. For example, on hydration, the personal actions could be
      i. simple: find and bring a water bottle to school;
      ii. moderate: replace sugary or caffeinated drinks with water; or
      iii. involved: measure water intake (as a liquid and in food) for a week.

6. *Jigsaw Sharing in Home Groups* (10 minutes): Reform back in home groups, where each expert presents their facts, questions, and actions in succession with the others.
7. *Lifeplay* (5 minutes): Debrief as a class for any further insights while still in home groups. Then invite every student to choose action(s) they will undertake personally; have them share their choice in their home group. Choose and share one as a teacher first.
8. *Accountability Home Groups* (5 minutes x 3–4 times): Every week or so, regroup to provide mutual support and accountability. It's important to emphasize themes of support and feedback, not just compare successes or failures, which can derail a group. Teachers can help this phase of the activity by defining the following terms: *authenticity, mutual support*, and *non-judgment*. Caution students against traits of competitiveness and criticism, but also inaction. Teachers can share their progress first, though students don't have to share, publicly or in the group. Structure time as follows:
    a. each student checks in, then shares how their personal action is going (optional);
    b. group brainstorming and problem-solving to support each other; and/or
    c. students can adjust their actions or choose another if the first one is going well.
9. *Integration Strategy*: Jigsaws are an incredible tool for curricular learning and building community in the classrooms. Use them over time in different ways (with visible random groupings) to build interdependence and student-centered learning. The trust level required drops when moving away from personal health into curricular areas.
10. *Schoolwide Extension*: Depending on space available, invite the class next door to join in the "wellness J.A.G.," making even more diverse groups and spreading wellness.
11. *Safety*: Students who struggle with any aspect of physical health can benefit from getting factual information and effective strategies in an open way, but keep in mind

students don't have to share personally about which quiz they took, or their chosen goal, if they choose to keep it private. Obesity is based on many complex factors, including body type biases. Focus on healthy lifestyle and body acceptance rather than weight loss.[7]

Keywords: caring, collaborative, choice, empower, foundational, integration, lifeplay, physical, restorative, schoolwide, social, support

Self-Care/Self-Love Playsheet

> "Self-care is never a selfish act—it is simply good stewardship of the only gift I have, the gift I was put on earth to offer others. Anytime we can listen to our true self and give it the care it requires, we do it not only for ourselves, but for the many others whose lives we touch."
>
> —Parker Palmer

Self-care wasn't actually a thing until 1981, when the National Library of Medicine defined it as "caring for self when ill." This illness-oriented definition was later broadened to "positive actions and adopting behaviors to prevent illness." Self-care, like well-being, is much more than illness care or prevention, bringing proactive self-love in every domain of wellness.

Since self-care has its roots in physical health, this activity is presented here, but it offers another opportunity to highlight the interconnectedness of whole-being. The activity works very well when used in conjunction with self-care acronyms (see supplements, p. 232).

Summary: Playfully explore some domains of wellness, including the physical.
Time: 10 minutes
Trust Required: Low

1. *Prep* (2 minutes): Copy handout 9.1 "Self-Care/Self-Love Playsheet" for the class.
2. *Play* (5 minutes): This is not a worksheet but a playsheet. Students and teachers play by:
   a. (perhaps) checking some things they are already doing, and smiling;
   b. (possibly) circling something that resonates, and noticing;
   c. (maybe) finding the emptiest column, and being grateful for space to grow; and/or
   d. (perchance) filling in some blanks with ideas, then doodling, and laughing.
3. *Debrief* (5 minutes): Students may share what they thought, felt, checked, circled, or filled in, but keep it light. This is an awareness-raising activity to be done with kindness, not self-judgment. Teachers sharing their own experience greatly improve student buy-in.
4. *Lifeplay*: Invite students to share what drew their attention on the playsheet and run with it in their lives for a few weeks. What are they already doing? What did they circle (as something to start doing) that resonated for them? Which column(s) are fullest or emptiest? Check in periodically and debrief to see how self-care is going.

Keywords: caring, cognitive, choice, creative, emotional, journal, lifeplay, physical, social, spiritual

Handout 9.1. Self-Care/Self-Love Playsheet

Name: _____

This is a playsheet, not a worksheet, so feel free to play by

- (perhaps) checking some things you are already doing, and smiling;
- (possibly) circling something that resonates, and noticing;
- (maybe) finding the emptiest column, and being grateful for space to grow; and/or
- (perchance) filling in some blanks with ideas, then doodling, and laughing.

Handout 9.1. (continued)

Emotional	Mental	Physical	Social	Spiritual
Taking a deep, abdominal breath each time you enter a new place/space.	Turning off devices for a spell here and there, and for a longer spell too.	Taking a walk or hike, riding a bike, swimming, or exercising.	Sharing feelings about an experience with a friend.	Connecting with nature, watching plants and animals grow and flow.
Using positive self-talk, and kindly noticing self-judgment.	Reading a book, journal, or magazine article, or the back of a cereal box.	Eating something healthy each meal, or just eating each meal.	Hugging someone (or asking for a hug) at least ten times a day for a week.	Concentrating with love on the flame of a candle, a flower, or your love.
Holding regular date nights with yourself.	Expressing your thoughts, feelings, and dreams in a journal.	Soaking in a bath or a long, hot shower, maybe with some candles.	Playing with, enjoying, and loving a pet.	Meditating, contemplating, and praying.
Singing, making sound, humming, or listening to music.	Making a to-do list, and accepting some things may not get done.	Eating mindfully: sitting, savoring, and undistracted.	Expressing and maintaining healthy boundaries from you-know-who.	Taking the shape and movement of birds, grass in the wind, or a cloud.
Watching children play and loving your inner child in a joyful way.	Writing a poem, a song, a positive social media post, a love letter.	Stretching and moving to music, dancing alone or in public.	Spending more time where you feel you belong, and less time where you don't.	Doing routines with absolute presence, devotion, and love.
Acknowledging your achievements, large and small.	Previewing your day upon awakening, and reviewing it upon retiring.	Practicing yoga, pilates, aerobics, or anything sweaty.	Expressing gratitude in person to someone good.	Listening to a guided meditation.
Taking responsibility, making restitution, expressing remorse, acknowledging impact.	Listening to free podcasts on drives, when walking, or when doing a chore.	Discerning when your body feels hungry versus thirsty versus stressed versus tired versus bored.	Calling or having a video chat with a long distance friend or relative.	Practicing a daily quiet time to connect to your inner world.

Handout 9.1. (continued)

Emotional	Mental	Physical	Social	Spiritual
Silently wishing good things for yourself	Making a list of short term and long term goals, and taking one small step.	Sitting in the sun for ten minutes or strolling in a garden or park.	Letting go of an unhealthy, unbalanced, or unloving relationship.	Visualizing yourself in a peaceful place, creating a safe haven internally.
Keeping an emotional journal, noticing and recording your feelings once a day.	Working on a puzzle, coloring, or other mentally soothing activity.	Tracking macronutrients for a week: carbohydrates, fat, protein.	Listening to one person per day with all your being, for as long as they want to share.	Doing something of service for others or for your community.
Feeling your fear and taking a positive risk for change.	Letting go of negative beliefs that limit your life, by Googling how to do that.	Taking stairs twice, standing at a computer, walking when on the phone.	Silently wishing good things for every person you meet, smiling warmly.	Joining a spiritual group or faith-based group that moves you.
Exercising, eating, and resting well when overly emotional.	Journaling mental stories, thoughts, reactions, and daydreams for a week.	Exploring sleep hygiene (less screens/caffeine, dark/quiet room).	Joining a peer support group or club or hobby or game group you love.	Learning about the beliefs of a faith you are unfamiliar with.
Seeing a therapist, social worker, or other mental health professional.	Listing your traits, needs and wants, or taking a personality test.	Seeing a professional: doctor, naturopath, nutritionist, chiropractor, etc.	Reaching out to a friend for a life chat or a support line when you need it	Studying with a spiritual teacher in person or watching free talks online.
Printing out an emotion wheel and circling how you feel on it for a week.	Practicing mindfulness formally or in little bits here and there.	Taking a nap when it feels right.	Nurturing relationships with loving others who make you feel good.	Reading about the wisdom of the ages in great spiritual works.

Sleep Hygiene Lab

> "There is no sunrise so beautiful that it is worth waking me up to see it."
>
> —Mindy Kaling

Bryan's favorite thing about Ms. Gauthier was something she often did with the kindies, but also did when she covered his grade-8 class. When things were dragging in the afternoon, or somebody was acting up, she would quietly say "Heads down please." Then the whole class would have to fold their arms on the desks and rest their heads on them. Bryan's smile never left his face while he closed his eyes to enjoy the precious few minutes, even after he fell asleep.

With a disrupted biological clock, chronic over-commitment, excessive screen time, and even sleep disorders, teens need much more than some "heads down" time. Grade 7–12 students require between eight and ten hours of sleep nightly, yet most high school students get fewer than seven hours, and up to 24 percent have insomnia disorders.[8]

Sleep doesn't get as much attention as diet or exercise in body-conscious teens, but it's an equally important pillar of the physical well-being trifecta. In fact, it may be the most important, since insufficient sleep increases hunger for foods that are not the best fuel, while good sleep has a beneficial effect on exercise and energy.[9] But the benefits of sleep stretch beyond the physical into almost every domain of well-being.

- *Safety:* sleep reduces the likelihood of high-risk behaviors, accidents, and alcohol use.
- *Cognitive:* sleep boosts attention, creativity, memory, and overall academic success.
- *Emotion:* sleep correlates to mood, emotional development, and mental health.
- *Physical*: sleep aids in body development, immune system health, weight loss, and more.
- *Resilience:* sleep reduces irritability and contributes to good decision making.
- *Social*: nobody likes a tired grump.

Students aren't the only sleepy ones in schools, 43 percent of teachers slept an average of six hours or less per night and experience more sleep problems than reported by the general population.[10] Students and teachers would both benefit from valuing sleep as much as diet or exercise. This sleep lab is an opportunity for everyone in the classroom to better understand sleep benefits, sleep hygiene, personal habits, and implement positive changes over time.

> **Summary**: Reflect on sleep hygiene and explore changes that can contribute to better rest.
> **Time**: 5–10 minutes × 7 classes over a period of weeks
> **Trust Required**: Low
>
> 1. *Prep* (2 minutes): Copy handout 9.2 "Sleep Hygiene Lab" for students and teacher.
> 2. *Reflect* (5 minutes): Have students complete parts A, B, and C of the reflection, filling in their totals under the "1st" tally. Scores need not be shared; they are for self-reflection.
> 3. *Debrief* (5 minutes): Hold a class discussion or circle to explore the following:
>   a. What stood out in doing the reflection?
>   b. What do we already know about sleep hygiene or the importance of sleep?
>   c. What's something you can do to improve sleep hygiene? (Students can make notes on part D of the handout.)
> 4. *Lifeplay*: Invite students to implement one or two changes over the next couple weeks, noting their changes in part E. As with the jigsaw (p. 214), teachers can create groups to build accountability and mutual support, or keep it as an individual exercise. Remind students once or twice a week about the lab and to bring it to class.
> 5. *Two Week Debrief* (10 minutes): After two weeks, debrief with students, being sure to share as a teacher yourself.

Complete A, B, and C again under the "2nd" heading. Use parts F and G to reflect on whether sleep hygiene intentions materialized, and if they had any impact. At this time, part H can be reviewed to provide additional ideas for students (in addition to the elements in A, B, and C). The class can also circle up and co-construct some best practices for sleep to add even more ideas. This builds knowledge of sleep hygiene over time as students repeatedly reconsider these elements.

6. *Four Week Debrief* (10 minutes): After four weeks, debrief again in a similar way, completing A, B, and C again under the "3rd" heading and using parts I and J to reflect. This process can be repeated as long as it is providing benefits. Changes may be difficult, but with time and patient effort a great deal can be done to improve sleep.

7. *Safety*: Some students may have sleep apnea, restless limbs, nightmares, or other sleep challenges. Sleep can be a sensitive area for some, so keep sharing optional, and post information (see p. 53) where additional support can be accessed if needed.

8. *Integration Strategy*: A sleep study could be integrated in biology, health, science, or mathematics, but there could be a creative connection in almost any subject. Free sleep tracking apps can provide additional data that may support curricular applications.

9. *Schoolwide Extension*: Inviting another class to join in the sleep study boosts synergy, engagement, and the spread of wellness.

Keywords: card, caring, cognitive, collaborative, choice, integration, journal, lifeplay, physical, safety, schoolwide, social

Handout 9.2

Sleep Hygiene Lab   Name: _____

A. *My Bedroom Space (20 points)*   1st 2nd 3rd
1) How comfortable is your mattress/pillow
   from 0 (awful) to 4 (super-comfy)?   ___ ___ ___
2) How cool is your room from 0 (warm/hot)
   to 4 (cooler than 67° F or 18° C)?   ___ ___ ___
3) How dark is your room from 0 (lit up) to
   4 (pitch black)?   ___ ___ ___
4) How quiet is where you sleep from 0 (noisy)
   to 4 (totally silent)?   ___ ___ ___
5) Interruptions (noises, pet visits, etc.) per
   night from 0 (many) to 4 (none)?   ___ ___ ___
                                          TOTAL ___ ___ ___

B. *My Daytime Habits (20 points)*   1st 2nd 3rd
Self-score with 0 (rarely), 1 (sometimes), 2 (half
the time), 3 (mostly), 4 (always/almost always).
  6) I wake up at the same time every day,
     including weekdays and weekends.   ___ ___ ___
  7) I get some good sunlight each day.   ___ ___ ___
  8) I am physically active during the day.   ___ ___ ___
  9) I don't smoke.   ___ ___ ___
 10) I avoid caffeine/energy drinks, especially
     in the afternoon and evening.   ___ ___ ___
                                          TOTAL ___ ___ ___

C. *My Evening Habits (20 points)*   1st 2nd 3rd
11) I don't eat big, heavy, or spicy meals or
    drink caffeine close to bedtime.   ___ ___ ___
12) I go to bed at the same time every night,
    including weekdays and weekends.   ___ ___ ___
13) I get 8–10 hours of sleep each night.   ___ ___ ___
14) I use a consistent routine (e.g., brush teeth,
    PJs, etc.) before going to bed.   ___ ___ ___
15) I don't look at screens one hour before
    I sleep and turn off my devices at night.   ___ ___ ___
                                          TOTAL ___ ___ ___

Reflection and Change Part 1   Date: _____

D. Which area(s) above had the highest or lowest totals? What are the most important factors that you feel affect your sleep? Did anything else stand out for you?

E. Record changes you could try over the next two weeks, along with the associated number from above. If you are changing wake-up or go-to-bed times, work in small steps.

\# _____ _____
\# _____ _____
\# _____ _____

Reflection and Change Part 2   Date: _____
                                    (two weeks later)

F. Redo parts A, B, and C under the 2nd heading. What, if anything, has changed about your sleep? Did you manage to make your changes totally, somewhat, or not at all? Change takes time and patience so have some self-compassion.

_____
_____
_____

G. Record a few changes you could try over the next couple weeks below. These could be the same as before or new ones. Again, if you are changing sleep/wake-up times, do it slowly.

\# _____ _____
\# _____ _____
\# _____ _____

Suggestions for Better Sleep

H. Here are some additional ideas to support your sleep which may work well together with any or all of the above. Make a note beside any of these that you would like to add to your sleep lab.

Have a warm shower or bath before bed. _____

Write in a paper journal or read a printed book before bed. _____

Listen to soft, soothing music, set to automatically shut off. _____

Practice deep breathing or meditation. _____

Have a light, healthy snack before bed. _____

Drink warm milk or herbal tea before bed. _____

Use earplugs and/or an eye cover. _____

Use a soothing (white) noise machine or app. _____

Reflection and Change Part 3   Date: _____
(four weeks later)

I. How have your changes gone; did you manage to keep your changes? It can be hard to adjust habits so give yourself time and dedication. What, if anything, has changed about your sleep?
_____
_____
_____

J. Record one or two changes (could be the same changes as before or new ones) you could try going forward. Again, if you are changing sleep/wake-up times, do it slowly.
_____
_____
_____

K. *Additional Reflections*
_____
_____
_____

SUPPLEMENTARIES: SHORT, SIMPLE, SAFE, OR SEARCHABLE PHYSICAL WELL-BEING

- *Circle Energizers* are fast and fun movements that can warm up a group, start a circle, or inject energy at any point in class. Debriefing is usually unnecessary as the energetic boost to participants is clear. See also *circle games* (p. 197), which are a little more involved but still fun. *Search terms*: circle, classroom, games, energizers.
    - *Dancing Circle* has a person dancing in the middle of a standing circle, with everyone else trying to imitate their moves (or doing their own thing). When the music skips to the next song (every fifteen seconds), the middle person invites somebody else to jump in and join them. Be sure to ask a few students to agree to get things going or start things off yourself as a teacher. Great for staff too.
    - *Toss Across* a ball, to another person in the circle, perhaps while calling their name or a greeting. Tell participants to remember who they tossed to, ensuring everyone gets the ball once, and then repeat the pattern again, seeing how fast they can go. Perhaps add a second ball and then a third that goes backward. Toss Across helps everyone learn names while having fun.
- *Classroom Ergonomics* pays attention to the furniture in the room and how students use their bodies (or not) when learning. Stand-up desks, ergonomic computer stations, small group stand-up whiteboards, adjustable furniture, and moveable (or motion) furniture can go a long way to helping bodies feel better (see p. 213 for more). *Search terms*: classroom, ergonomics.
- *Elvish Sleep* is an activity that fits after an extended period of hard work, completion of a significant task in class, or just because it's needed. Lower the lights and invite students to lay on yoga mats or carpets with eyes closed or just put their heads down on desks. Either way, students won't wonder if anyone can see them if everyone's eyes are closed. Play a guided meditation or nature sounds for 10 or 15 minutes, allowing for deep relaxation. Students may have waking dreams like Tolkien's elves while others may actually fall asleep—both are okay. Given the incredibly positive impact of rest, and its related impact on safety, this could be a most effective use of classroom time.

- *Mindful Eating* reminds students that food is so much more than fuel. Offer students a raisin, baby carrot, or chocolate (choice is best) that they place on a clean sheet of paper. Invite them through the stages below for 10 to 30 seconds per stage:
  - look at, smell, and feel the food without holding it;
  - hold the food, and see, smell, and feel it again;
  - listening to the body, discern if there is hunger for this food (if not, stop here);
  - put the food on the lips and tip of tongue, just feeling and tasting it;
  - put the food in the mouth, not chewing but just holding;
  - chew slowly, moving the food to different parts of the tongue;
  - swallow slowly in small bites; and
  - close the eyes and feel the body.

  The debrief could get into listening to the body, as young children do by only eating when they are hungry. Ask if students eat on a schedule, whether they are hungry or not? Debrief the purposes of food beyond fuel, such as making good feelings, providing a sensory experience, sharing meals that bring people together, reflecting traditions, or sharing diverse cultures. Invite students to try mindful eating and intuitive eating for lifeplay. *Search terms*: mindful eating, intuitive eating.
- *N.E.A.T.* is non-exercise activity thermogenesis, a way to increase movement and boost energy by doing regular daily tasks other than exercise (also see "Walk the Talk," p. 206). Even trivial activities such as chewing or fidgeting can significantly raise metabolism, and activities that don't require gyms, special shoes, or equipment are also more accessible.[11] Students and teachers can get creative here, brainstorming NEAT ideas, and keeping a "NEAT-meter" on the board to capture new ideas and accomplishments:
  - Taking an extra hallway, or stairway up and down, when moving in the school
  - Parking in a distant spot (rather than the closest) or getting off one stop early
  - Automatically getting up and walking around whenever checking a phone

- Standing up while working on a computer placed on a shelf or standing station
- Making sedentary pleasures like gaming a reward after some activity
- Do sit-ups for every 30 minutes of watching a screen
- *Physical Well-Being Apps* abound, are constantly changing, and some of them are actually very useful! Apps supporting the physical domain can track (steps, macronutrients, hydration, or sleep), train (aerobics, exercise, or yoga), and more. As with the jigsaw (p. 214), students research in small groups to find age-appropriate apps for the wellness areas in which the class is interested. These can be shared for a joint experience or left to student choice in support of many wellness efforts. *Search terms*: teenage, youth, app, [diet, exercise, etc.]
- *Pillar Quizzes* are online quizzes for youth on various topics within the pillars of physical well-being. Give quiz links to students, some time to complete them, and have a quick debrief. What myths were debunked? What new information was learned? Most importantly, what did students learn about themselves? *Search terms*: youth, [blank], quiz (where [blank] is a pillar keyword, such as: exercise, macronutrients, sleep, hydration, hygiene, etc.).
- *Self massage* soothes nerves and releases tension for a mental refresh. Probing with fingertips is a welcome start, adjusting pressure and feeling which area of the body has tension. Having a few different balls (e.g., tennis, lacrosse) or a roller always available lets students self-destress without interrupting class. *Search terms*: self massage.
- *Stretches and exercises* boost mental focus and flexibility to balance extended sitting in class. A huge variety of warmups, moves, and cooldowns can be found, whether standalone or using classroom desks and chairs. Start simple and build as comfort grows. *Search terms*: stretch/exercise/yoga, chair/desk/office.
- *Gains and Drains* is a brainstorm where students and the teacher complete a T-chart with the heading "gains" (what fills me up) and "drains" (what depletes me). The subject could be anything wellness-related: exercise, food, and more. Debrief with a bit of lifeplay:

- What did you notice? What would you like to see more of, or less of, in your life?
- Did you think of any gains or drains that are *not* currently a part of your life? If not, write some down. What does thinking of these do for you, if anything?
- Going forward, what can you say "yes" or "no" to?
- *Self-Care/Love Acronyms* combine personally relevant aspects of well-being into a powerful reminder word. A teacher might put their C.A.P. on before every class (calm, aware, present) or a student might H.A.L.T. before entry to check whether they are *hungry, anxious, lonely,* or *tired* to give themselves what they most need. Creating the acronym oneself adds personal meaning, and it can change as life changes. *Search terms*: word, finder.
  - D.R.E.A.M.Y. = daylight, rest, elevate, appreciate, mindfulness, yoga.
  - CFP 532 = a license to eat well: carbs, fats, and protein in a 5:3:2 calorie ratio.
  - R.E.P.E.A.T. = reps, exercise, protein, elongate, asleep (by) ten.
  - S.H.A.P.E.D. = sleep, hydrate, authenticity, practice/exercise, diet.
- *Take a Stand* makes meetings, small group work, and one-on-one interactions more active by having everyone stand rather than sit. Standing is a welcome change for most people, is incredibly simple to implement, and reduces sedentary seated time.[12] Moreover, interactions tend to be more efficient when standing.[13] Having standing desks or tables is ideal, but getting creative with chart stands, white boards, window ledges, and mobile devices can work wonders. *Search terms*: standing meetings.
- *Take Five Movement Breaks* are short, movement-based breaks for use in any class, assembly, or school group. Movement breaks validate daily physical activity, taking breaks, and having fun. Move furniture and bags out of the way as needed, or go outside if possible to increase focus and provide a little hallway informal chat time with students on the way. *Search terms*: classroom, body, physical, activity, movement, breaks.
  - *1, 2, 3, 4* has students in pairs facing each other, with somebody (not the teacher, who is paired up) calling out a number 1

through 4. One is left hand high five, two is right hand high five, three is right foot tap, and four is left foot tap.
- *Head, Shoulders, Knees, and Toes . . . and PEN!* has pairs facing each other with a pen (or any toy or ball) on a desk beside them (not the floor, lest they conk heads). A caller randomly calls out the words *heads, shoulders, knees,* or *toes* (with the usual movements), and when they say "PEN!" both players try to grab the pen. Swap the order of the words, repeat them, and speed up until confusion and laughter result.
- *Name Your Move* invites each person to create a movement or action that starts with the first letter of their name, such as "Corrine Cross Country Skiing" or "Scott Squats." Each person demonstrates their move, then everyone repeats it while saying the name. Go around again faster for a sure laugh.
- *Over and Under* has students in lines of equal length, facing the same way, jogging on the spot. The front student passes a ball or toy to the person behind overhead, who passes it behind under the legs, and so on. The last person runs with the object to the front and starts passing again. Repeat until everyone has run up. Teachers can participate to make even numbers or just because they need it too.
- *Rock, Paper, Scissors Grand Tournament* starts with pairs competing in a best of three rock, paper, scissors rounds. Whoever wins is followed around and cheered on by all the people they beat. Winners hold up their hands to find a new challenger for each round. Be warned, or thrilled, that some serious noise can be generated, especially if teachers join in.

10

SPIRITUAL WELL-BEING

Transcendence, Union, and Peace

"The inner life of . . . young people is intimately bound up with matters of meaning, purpose, and connection, with creative expression and moments of joy and transcendence. All these qualities are central to both emotional intelligence and to constructively filling the spiritual void.

Classroom environments that acknowledge and invite such experiences help students break down stereotypes, improve discipline, increase academic motivation, foster creativity, and keep more kids in school."[1]

—Rachael Kessler

The origin of the word spirit is *breath*: an invisible essence of life. Putting spirituality into words is like capturing the breath: portraying a cloud of notions that inherently defies depiction, yet billows to touch every domain of well-being and beyond:[2]

- Peace, bliss, or love, beyond everyday experience (emotional)
- The discovery of ultimate meaning by finding our essential nature (eudaimonia)
- Communion—and union—with the whole of the natural world (environmental)

- Oneness in a sacred relationship with another person or all of life (social)
- Transcendent, harmonious flow that merges with life (cognitive, physical)
- The dropping of all resistance, having no "self" to fight against, or for (resilience)
- Absolute presence or emptiness in the silent abiding of the present moment
- Worship or communion with the supreme, divine, ultimate, or infinite
- The experience of non-separateness—a wholeness with all

As inscrutable and diverse as spirituality may be, it is just as compelling. Approximately 85 percent of people worldwide identify with any one of thousands of religions. Many more explore secular contemplative practices in uniquely personal ways.[3] A 2003 survey of six thousand youth around the world, spanning eight countries and five continents, revealed a broad spectrum of religiosity, spirituality, atheism, and secularity.[4] Across all these identities, the majority pursue spiritual development in many of the ways described above without adhering strongly to a religion.

Whether a teacher identifies as religious, spiritual, or neither, and whether a school is faith-based or secular, it is vital to acknowledge and respect the spiritual life. While teachers do not advance religious doctrine outside of faith-based schools, they can nourish the basic human freedom of belief and manifest that belief in different ways.[5]

These diverse ways of living the infinite and the everyday share some common essences: *transcendence*, *union*, and *peace*.[6] Such essences are universal in bringing people to the summits of well-being, whether they are agnostic, freethinking, humanist, religious, secular, or spiritual.[7] For adolescents, connecting to others, nature, the transcendent, and self brings joy and other benefits.[8] Yet it's not just majesty or mystery that transports us, it can also be travesty and tragedy.

Shamil flipped on the classroom lights to find the desks and chairs in the precise configuration of chaos they held at 3:05 p.m. the afternoon before. It was early in the morning, early in the semester, and early in his teaching career. The administration had given him a dog's breakfast timetable that included the most difficult-to-reach students. He had happily worked long and hard to become a teacher, but the daily grind of fighting classroom fires was draining him—mind, heart, body, and soul. The school day hadn't even started, but he already felt spent. He knelt to pick up a chair, but instead he put one hand to the floor and one to his forehead.

The words came then, his voice soft, low, and clear: expressing gratitude for being alive that morning; giving thanks to every student by name; for the gift of being their teacher; appreciating their parents for trusting young lives into his care; blessing ancestors for their faith that he would pour water on the seeds they had planted. Shamil saw himself then as a teacher, a student, a parent, and an ancestor: *becoming* them all at once. As he came back to the room, he knew he could love them again. Standing up slowly, he quietly set the first chair back on its feet.

With any transcendent experience, there may be a feeling of union or merging. When the personal sense of being a separate self dissolves, a deeper "self" emerges that is an expression of an indivisible whole. Whereas connection implies a linking of two separate things, union discovers—or rediscovers—oneness, bringing great peace. In contact with unparalleled beauty, vast scale, or the incomprehensible, this can crest into awe.[9] As such, any one essence brings all of them. A tree in the wind that captivates, an unspoken bond with a beloved, the vastness of the night sky—all these stop us in our tracks, while simultaneously launching us. In such times, the fullness of here and now unites with the beyond.

This unity has been described by artists, emperors, and computer engineers:

- "I believe that what people call God is something in all of us."—John Lennon
- "Meditate often on the interconnectedness and mutual interdependence of all things in the universe."[10]—Marcus Aurelius
- "You are never alone. You are eternally connected with everyone."[11]—Amit Ray

Transcendence and union (if not peace) may seem metaphysical to some or of little practical use in school. Yet out of these spring freedom, serenity, and love. A classroom willing to explore them opens doors to meaning, fulfillment, and a deep oneness with the world. As the personal self is transcended, learning and well-being flow (p. 163) as every thought, word, and action is rooted in love. Educators may only dream of such a classroom, yet to acknowledge that it can be a reality, and not just a dream, is the first courageous and powerful step.

These activities explore transcendence, connection, or peace with students. Whether navigating them within the theme of spirituality or wellness, acknowledging and accepting every unique spirit in the classroom brightens everyone's flame. In this way, the domain of spiritual well-being—the breath that is the source of life, and the life beyond—can be illuminated.

Key Messages

- Spiritual life can be experienced in any number of ways, some of which relate to other well-being domains, and some which explore domains beyond everyday life.
- Most young people express their spirituality without strong ties to a religion, whether they identify as being part of a religion or not.
- Transcendence, union, and peace are universal human experiences that connect strongly to well-being, and are often experienced together.
- Acknowledging individual beliefs and lived experiences is crucial to spiritual well-being.

SPIRITUAL WELL-BEING ACTIVITIES

Contemplative Practices (Main Move)

> "The personal changes that often occur with regular contemplative practice, such as increased patience, compassion, and concentration, can play a part in the positive transformation of individuals, organizations, and social institutions."[12]
>
> —Maia Duerr

SPIRITUAL WELL-BEING

In 2002, Maia Duerr led a research project to catalog the proliferation of contemplative practices around the world. To represent the growth and branching of these diverse practices, the image of a tree naturally came to her. Her colleague Carrie Bergman provided a visual representation, and the *Tree of Contemplative Practices* was born. The tree is freely available for education in a variety of formats from the Center for Contemplative Mind in Society.[13]

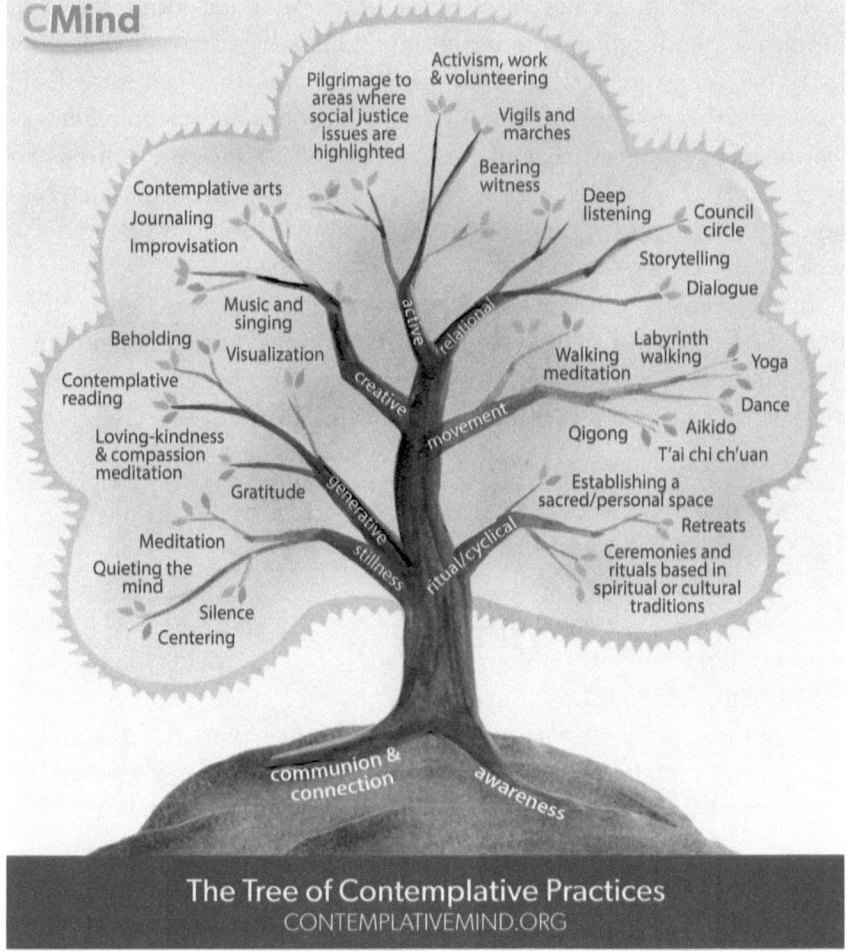

Figure 10.1. Tree of Contemplative Practices
Source: CMind. (2021). The Tree of Contemplative Practices [Illustration]. The Center for Contemplative Mind in Society. https://www.contemplativemind.org/practices/tree

Contemplative practices develop awareness, empathy, compassion, and self-regulation, while directly exploring the nature of consciousness.[14] The vast majority of these practices require no ties to religious or spiritual traditions, though some have ties to various faiths.

Traditional practices like yoga or meditation are included, but so too are reading, singing, or walking a mindful labyrinth. As a secular and inclusive model, the tree is ideal for classroom use, reflecting the diversity of the secular, the spiritual, or the religious everywhere.

Saki Santorelli, former director of the Center for Mindfulness in Medicine (the original school for mindfulness-based stress reduction [MBSR]) refers to the transcendence and union that can arise from contemplative practices: "Contemplative practices help people learn—via direct experience—that the self is less like a noun and more like a verb. . . . In the process, what one thinks of as 'me' becomes much bigger. This 'enlarging' alters your relationship with self, others, and the world, irrevocably."[15]

In this activity, students and teachers explore contemplative practices, finding out what they already enjoy and maybe trying new ones. As awareness and connectedness take root, contemplative practitioners awaken to the possibility of multiple domains of wellness.

> **Summary**: Explore a range of contemplative practices.
> **Time**: 5–10 minutes × 4
> **Trust Required**: Low
>
> 1. *Prep* (5 minutes): Share the tree by making copies, sharing a link, or projecting it in class.
> 2. *Climbing* (5 minutes): Invite students to explore the tree and find practices that resonate for them. They can do a little research if desired. This exploration can be done in small groups, but individual reflection is an essential foundation to begin contemplative practices. Invite whole group sharing of what was discovered and discuss the common elements of awareness and connection on the trunk as well as the branch categories.

3. *Lifeplay* (10 minutes): Invite students to choose a contemplative practice to commit to explore for a period of a few weeks. To prime the contemplative pump, some class time may be given to explore a particular practice (or two). This book details several of these including journaling (p. 172), gratitude (p. 199), mindfulness (p. 145), and deep listening (p. 70). Teachers, as always, participate fully with students.
4. *Grafting* (5 minutes): Students can add new practices to the tree, or even new categories. Anything done with sincerity and sacredness can make it contemplative. Be open to diverse ideas; flower arranging may work for one student, while another may prepare food for loved ones. Even mindful hugs can be an expression of contemplation.
5. *Debrief* (5 minutes × 2): Periodically check in and invite sharing around what happened with the contemplative practices lifeplay. Encourage the sharing of experiences, thoughts, and feelings, as well as the impact of contemplation in different forms. Look for evidence of transcendence, union, or peace in the debrief.
6. *Integration Strategy*: Consider inviting local experts to lead the class in particular practices that are relevant to the subject area. For example, a visual artist for an arts class or a dance or Tai Chi instructor for physical education.
7. *Safety*: Participating in and sharing contemplative, spiritual, or faith-based practices is always invitational and optional. The tree naturally provides choice, allowing students to find areas of personal comfort and security, rather than feeling pushed in any direction.

Keywords: caring, cognitive, choice, creative, emotional, foundational, gratitude, identity, integration, journal, lifeplay, mindfulness, outdoor, physical, social, spiritual

Death Dialogues: Questions to Ask Before Dying

> "Schools should be the place where [students] learn about death and dying as part of the curriculum. . . . The sooner we learn to accept this the better we will live with each other each day as we will acknowledge that we live in the shadow of our dying."[16]
>
> —Ethel King-McKenzie

Jacqueline put down the phone, called for the vice principal, and pinched her eyes shut. She could still hear the anguished voice of Tyler's mother telling her he had succumbed to his injuries. The crash had killed three teens, yet Tyler was the only one from her school. Jacqueline felt thankful for that, then guilty, and then just awful. She began drafting the letter to go home, as the vice principal called for extra social workers. As Jacqueline made a note to put the flag at half-mast, and tell Tyler's teachers in person, she realized all her personal problems had become very small.

Any death in a school community is sad, but premature ones are a tragedy. In a Zen parable, the words "father dies, son dies, grandson dies" are given as a blessing of gratitude for the natural order of dying. While we can't know the order or manner of our death, the fact that we will die one is one of life's few certainties. Another is the reluctance most people have to face this fact or even talk about it. In education, this has manifested in a century of learning about the beginnings of life (through sex education) without including the ends.

The absence of death education leaves students impacted by the death of pets, family members, or a loss at school allowing little or no opportunities to talk about it. While schools offer grief counseling in the wake of tragedies, few take up the offer. Caregivers may not talk with teens about deaths that occur, barred by their own grief or hoping to protect them from the same suffering. In any case, not discussing death reinforces its taboo.

Talk about dying as a part of living. A growing awareness of organ donation, medical assistance in dying, living wills, and more makes death education for teens even more relevant, including a consideration of spiritual perspectives.[17] Without such learning, bereaved youth are at risk for substance use, depression, PTSD, and suicidal ideation—making death education potentially critical for well-being.[18]

Grade 7–12 students can understand and explore abstract concepts around death, along with its philosophical or spiritual questions. The questions in this activity open the door to that exploration as an ongoing discourse, not just after a death. Such conversations may initially bring discomfort, but health professionals and researchers have called for educators to have them.[19]

While death may hold grief, uncertainty, fear, and sometimes feel so pointless, it holds out one possibility at least—to illuminate the meaning in life. Stephen Jenkinson, spiritual activist and author of *Die Wise*,[20] conveys this truth: "The endings of life give life's meanings a chance to show. The beginning of the end of our order, our way, is now in view. This isn't punishment, any more than dying is a punishment for being born. Instead, the world whispers: All we need of you is that you be human, now."

Summary: Discuss death and end of life with students.
Time: 10 minutes per dialogue
Trust Required: High

1. *Safety*: The intention of these dialogues is to help young people understand and accept death as a part of life, and to normalize conversations about dying. The following considerations can create a safer space for students to explore and share their feelings.
    a. *Not* talking about death may have an adverse impact on students, who could experience the death of a loved one (premature or not) traumatically, or respond to it in other unhealthy ways.
    b. Consider giving a content warning prior to a discussion, and provide accommodations, support, or alternatives for those who want them.
    c. Look for natural entry points to open a discussion, such as the death of a famous person, or news about end-of-life

legislation. If a school death has occurred, follow the direction of professional support staff in helping students.
   d. Spread these questions out over different times, perhaps discussing one (or at most a few) at a time, rather than having a single, prolonged discussion of more of them.
   e. Answer student questions honestly, and avoid euphemisms such as "gone to sleep," instead using accurate terms such as "died."
   f. It is natural and okay to not know the answers to any or all of these questions. Be open to not knowing, and let students know you don't know all the answers.
2. *Circle* (10 minutes): Gauge how students are feeling by taking refuge (p. 17) and doing a group check-in, then pose one or more questions below non-sequentially (see p. 61).
   a. There are many euphemisms (or substitutes) for words like death, dead, or dying, such as "passed on" or "gone to sleep." Why do you think this is?
   b. Why do most people seem to not want to talk about death?
   c. Have you registered for organ donation? Why or why not?
   d. What is the medical definition of death? How does this relate to defining life?
   e. What might a person experiencing the death of a loved one think or feel?
   f. What might a person dying themselves think or feel?
   g. Grief is a healthy response to a big loss. What are some ways people express grief; what stages do they experience? Why do people express grief so differently?
   h. If a friend was grieving or bereaved, how might you support them?
   i. What do you know about death? What would you like to know? Has anyone had a near-death experience?
   j. If you knew you were going to die in a year, would you change anything? Consider relationships or goals you might want to resolve in some way.

k. What preferences or decisions might you want for your own end of life? Consider palliative care (care that minimizes suffering for the dying), do-not-resuscitate orders, living wills, or medical assistance in dying (provide a glossary). How do people make these preferences known to those close to them?
l. Have you ever had to think about death? What did you think about it?
m. Does thinking and talking about death give you a different perspective on life? Consider beliefs, experiences, gratitude, regrets, relationships, and legacy.
n. Do you have any notions of what happens after death?
o. What is the meaning of death? How does death give meaning to life?

3. *Debrief*: The discussion itself is the debrief. Responses will get at thoughts, feelings, opinions, and wonderings around death and its impact on life.
4. *Integration Strategy*: Use curricular ties to death and dying as natural entry points, such as interpreting signs and symbols around death in art, reducing injury or death in safety talks, significant historical deaths, or other connections in social studies.
5. *Lifeplay*: Invite students to continue discussions with supportive others as they wish.

Keywords: caring, circle, emotional, eudaimonia, gratitude, integration, resilience, restorative, spiritual, support

Interbeing through Gazing

"Interbeing is the understanding that nothing exists separately from anything else. We are all interconnected. By taking care of another person, you take care of yourself."

—Thích Nhất Hạnh

Eye contact is often fleeting, and it can be difficult for many people, but it builds trust, intimacy, and emotional understanding.[21] Meeting the gaze also makes us seem more believable, confident, and intelligent to others.[22] When the eyes meet, they offer presence, social cues, emotional connection, and ultimately, a window to the soul.

Gazing is a form of partner meditation in which eye contact is made in silence for an extended period of time. This connection activates conscious and autonomic cognitive processes, as well as stimulating the amygdala.[23] Gazing can also lead to interconnectedness, communion, and *interbeing* (a term coined by Thích Nhất Hạnh, Zen teacher, peace activist, and writer).

It takes equanimity and sensitivity for two people to sit quietly and gaze into each other's eyes in silence. But with time and awareness, the fundamental essence of each person can be revealed and shared, leading to moments of deep connection and even transcendence.

> **Summary**: Make eye contact with oneself or a partner in silence, noticing what arises.
> **Time**: 2–10+ minutes
> **Trust Required**: Medium
>
> 1. *Explanation* (2 min.): Let students know they are going to pair up and gaze, which is to look into each other's eyes in silence. Encourage students to gaze with a partner, and they may also use their phone camera to self-gaze, or just sit in silent mediation if they prefer. Make visible, random partners and invite them to sit opposite their partner. Join in as a teacher if there are odd numbers. Describe gazing, perhaps using this suggested script:
>
>   > "When I start the 30-second timer, make natural eye contact with your partner and simply notice what arises. There's no need to think about what's happening, though thoughts will likely come. When they do come, just don't get absorbed in them and keep gazing. The main thing to

remember is to *notice what arises*. It's okay to blink or shift your gaze between the eyes, but to try to maintain eye contact as best they can without looking away."

2. *Gazing* (1–5 min.): Start the timer and cue students to gaze. After 30 seconds, invite them to close their eyes and self-reflect. They can then repeat gazing with new random partners as time allows or until it feels like time to debrief. Consider increasing or decreasing the gazing time based on comfort levels.
3. *Circle Gazing* (5 min, optional): Instead of being seated in chairs, students can stand in two concentric circles (see *fishbowl*, p. 190) with the inside circle facing the outside circle. Gazing pairs are formed between two people across from each other, with the teacher joining in. After each 30-second interval the outer circle rotates one person clockwise.
4. *Debrief* (5 minutes): After gazing, students can have individual reflection or notetaking time. Use the standard debrief questions, asking "What arose for you while gazing?" instead of "What happened?" Sometimes gazing will produce deep feelings or insights, sometimes no debrief will be needed. Be open to different possibilities.
5. *Safety*: For some people, eye contact can imply interest or dominance. For others, averting the gaze could be a sign of deference or respect. Students who do not wish to gaze for any reason may use their phones to self-gaze or meditate silently.
6. *Lifeplay*: Invite students to explore the impact of eye contact in different life situations. Debrief periodically when there is something to share.

Keywords: cognitive, circle, emotional, get-to-know, lifeplay, mindfulness, prep-free, restorative, social, spiritual

Unselfing (Guided Meditation)

"The most beautiful experience we can have is the mysterious. It is the fundamental emotion that stands at the cradle of true art and true science. Whoever does not know it and can no longer wonder, no longer marvel, is as good as dead, and his eyes are dimmed."

—Albert Einstein

Most people live life wrapped up in their "self": immersed in personal thoughts, bodies, and to-dos. This guided meditation invites a progressive unwrapping of these layers. In leaving the many layers of the self behind, there may be a taste of the self-transcendence. At a minimum, just considering what we are holding onto may loosen our grip, opening us to the possibility of release, and the intangible beyond.

> **Summary**: Progressively let go of different aspects of the self and debrief the experience.
> **Time**: 20 minutes
> **Trust Required**: Medium
>
> 1. *Centering* (2 minutes): Invite students to get comfortable in their seats or lying on mats (if available) with eyes closed. Dim the lights a little if desired. Tell students you will be guiding them through a short journey, and all they need to do is relax and visualize.
> 2. *Guided meditation* (10 minutes): Read this script, inserting pauses of a few seconds or more where shown and adjusting as feels natural for you.
>   a. *Eyes closed, notice your breathing, without needing to change it or have any thoughts. Give yourself this time to relax and just breathe* (pause). *Notice your body, feeling whatever is there* (pause). *Let everything be, and just chill* (pause).
>   b. *Now imagine a plain wooden door in front of you* (pause). *On the door your name is printed* (pause). *If you choose, you can walk through this door and leave your name*

behind (pause). *Open the door now and pass through (pause). Rest in the experience of leaving your name behind (pause).*
c. *Past the door you see a large, well-built chest (pause). As you approach it, consider everything you own: clothes, gear, books, . . . all your stuff (pause). If you like, place it all in this chest, which can hold everything easily (pause). When you have left behind all that you own, close the chest and move on (pause). Rest in the experience of leaving possessions behind (pause).*
d. *Up ahead you see a wall of hooks. On the hooks you can hang up your roles and responsibilities—all the hats you wear (pause). On one hook you can hang up being a student (pause). On others you can leave behind being a sister . . . brother . . . son . . . daughter . . . friend . . . worker . . . volunteer (pause). Leave all your roles and responsibilities on the hooks and pass by (pause). Rest in the experience of leaving your roles and responsibilities behind (pause).*
e. *Now another wall appears, with many cubby holes (pause). If you wish, here you can leave aspects of your identity: your age . . . gender . . . nationality . . . beliefs (pause). Store away in the cubbies everything you wish to, then turn away and move on (pause). Rest in the experience of leaving your identity behind (pause).*
f. *The way ahead is misty, with a comfortable chair rising from the mist (pause). If you like, you can rest here (pause). Feel your body sinking into the chair (pause). When you move on, you can leave your body safely behind (pause). Leave this place now, and leave your body as well (pause). Rest in the experience of being without your body (pause).*
g. *Up ahead is total blackness, but floating there is an empty crystal globe, sparkling and turning slowly (pause). Into this globe you can pour all your thoughts and memories, as well as anything else you still haven't let go of, and wish to (pause). Empty your mind completely now, along with*

everything else (pause). *Let it all go* (pause). *When you are ready, move on into the blackness* (pause). *Rest here for a while* (pause). [Let participants linger in this place for a minute or two in silence]

h. *Now, if you choose, you may turn around slowly, and go back* (pause). *See the crystal globe, shining with your thoughts and memories* (pause). *If you wish, take some time now to reclaim these* (pause). *Or you may simply continue* (pause).

i. *See the chair, with your body resting in it* (pause). *If you wish, you may inhabit your body again* (pause). *Or you may simply continue* (pause).

j. *See the walls of hooks and cubby holes, with all your roles, responsibilities, and identity* (pause). *If you wish, you may assume these again* (pause). *Or you may simply continue* (pause).

k. *See the chest ahead, with all your things in it* (pause). *If you wish, you may pick these up again* (pause). *Or you may simply continue* (pause).

l. *See the door ahead, with your name on it* (pause). *If you wish, you may open the door, and take your name back* (pause). *Or you may simply continue* (pause).

m. *Notice your breathing again, without needing to change it or have any thoughts. Give yourself this time to reflect* (pause). *Notice whatever is there* (pause).

3. *Debrief* (8 minutes): Students may be in a deeper, contemplative state so give some time for personal reflection and note-taking or journaling. Use the standard debrief (p. 13) and ask which aspects of the journey stood out? Which felt good, or difficult, to let go of? Was there any aspect of the self you would rather not reclaim? What might it be like to live with a less solid sense of self? Is the self fixed, or can it evolve or change?

4. *Safety*: Students may not wish to let go of certain fundamental aspects of their identity, so it is important to keep the language invitational, rather than directive.
5. *Lifeplay*: Invite students to experiment with evoking the feelings from the meditation throughout their day, noticing how that may change their interactions.

Keywords: cognitive, eudaimonia, identity, journal, lifeplay, mindfulness, prep-free, spiritual

SUPPLEMENTARIES: SHORT, SIMPLE, SAFE, OR SEARCHABLE SPIRITUAL WELL-BEING

- *Deeper Questions* starts by inviting students to think of any life situation or question, especially one that holds some degree of mystery. They then ask a question about it, perhaps starting with *why*. They then jot down a few possible responses to this first question. Pick one of these responses and a related second question. Repeat, perhaps up to five times or more. An example: "Why is this class so hard? Why do I care so much about school? Why do my parents care so much about grades? What happened to my parents to make them so grade-focused? Do I really have to feel the same way? What do I actually deeply care about?"
- *Human Being or Human Doing?* Kurt Vonnegut said he was the former, and not the latter. Some people are hyper-busy and trying to constantly achieve, others are so passive they aren't really living. Circle up with students and ask if they have an inclination to do or to be? How does that balance change in their lives? What do families or the media value most: doing or being? *Search terms*: human being or human doing.

ALL IS WELL

Awakening to the interconnectedness of life is also an ultimate realization of well-being. This shift happened for Thomas Merton (monk, mystic, and author) while running errands on a busy street: *"I was suddenly overwhelmed with the realization that I loved all these people, that they were mine and I theirs, that we could not be alien to one another even though we were total strangers. It was like waking from a dream of separateness."*[1] This waking up makes beloved of strangers, and beginnings of ends. Seeing the unity of life also reveals that thriving is deeply shared. Each drop of our personal well-being lifts the world, and the world lifts us in return. With this extraordinary union as our truest nature, the only question is how deeply we can awaken to it in schools.

Our collective survival depends on answering this question. Failing to awaken to our oneness with others and the Earth perpetuates "othering" and environmental destruction. Realizing that we are an inclusive whole makes such harmful actions unthinkable. Teachers must travel with students to the heart of this realization—that *we* can be well only if *all* are well—because classrooms are microcosms of the whole, as well as its future.

Awakening to wholeness might seem a lofty outcome, but it draws closer, and is more brightly illumined, with every wellness step taken.

As this book began with the following questions of well-being, this end becomes another beginning: an invitation for teachers and students to live these questions and find their own answers.

If success is chasing happiness, wealth, and status, then why does that feel so unwell? Traditional success isn't inherently bad. Fun, fortune, and fame might be unhealthy as singular obsessions, but they add to wellness when in balance with other domains. Success isn't wrong, but it needs to include other forms of wellness beyond material gains, and be inclusive of those who face unjust barriers, and do not share in that success equally.

Is well-being simply the absence of illness, is it mental health, or something else entirely? With at least nine domains, well-being is clearly much more than mental. The story of human development has been largely cognitive and physical. Yet burgeoning mental growth and technological proliferation has brought unchecked consumption, competition, and conquest. A lack of corresponding emotional development, and the psychological separation of people into groups, has contributed to othering, bias, and incalculable harm. As this splitting is contrary to the nature of interconnectedness, it threatens the health of all natural life.

For wellness to be deep and lasting for all, it must go beyond self-help, and even helping others, to reflect the union we are together. Well-being has to become a triumph of heart and soul as well as mind and body, broadening and brightening to include meaning-making, nature relatedness, social harmony, emotional thriving, flourishing in adversity, and self-transcendence.

Is baseline wellness fixed for life, or are there ways to change it? Curriculum documents are filled with thousands of cognitive standards, but very few teach students to love all three of their brains: head, heart, and gut. Mindfulness, self-directed neuroplasticity, and flow states change these brains for the good, for good. By deepening awareness, and tilting the cognitive spiral upward, they also nourish every domain of well-being with lasting, positive change.

Well-being was born of its bottom half: a response to unwellness that has resulted in detailed catalogs of every physical illness (ICD-11) and mental disorder (DSM-V) imaginable.[2] These responses help those in need get to a neutral baseline of health. But we can also bask in the upper half of well-being: a rising sun of flourishing. Positive wellness is wondrous for its own sake, prevents problems before they happen, and grows traits of well-being throughout life.

How can well-being be integrated with learning in classrooms and schools? The cross-curricular activities and integration strategies in this book are one response to this question. Teachers who develop a well-being expertise to match their subject knowledge will find even more powerful ways to integrate wellness. This proficiency comes through full teacher participation in well-being: living personal wellness that is shared with students.

How can wellness be social: developed collaboratively and shared for the greater good? Can the school community and world beyond benefit from classroom well-being? True wellness isn't personal, as the only separation of self and other is in the mind. Teachers who embrace well-being do so not just for students, or themselves, or even the "strangers" that their efforts touch in unknowable ways, but for everyone. As students begin thriving, their goodness is broadcast outward. The inherently communal nature of well-being then spreads in classrooms, schools, and connections that reach around the globe.

While this sharing is inevitable, it can be helped along by the lifeplay and schoolwide extensions in the activities. Sharing wellness cards (p. 263) plants even more seeds, as do the achievements (p. 259). Educators who lead wellness efforts in their schools and districts can do even more, sharing and building a pedagogy of flourishing throughout the profession.

Could the ultimate aim of public education shift to a union of learning and well-being? A powerful expression of unity is the embracing of well-being *as* learning (rather than *instead of* learning, or *in addition to* learning). Well-being pioneers make this happen in their classrooms, creating a seamless flow of learning and wellness. But for many, curriculum shifts will need to light the way forward. When both instruction and assessment of well-being are mandated, the line between learning and wellness is blurred. Ultimately, progress in human thriving in every domain will join academic achievement of traditional school subjects at the heart of learning.

School leaders help by approving and supporting well-being efforts, but they do even more by embodying wellness *as* leadership. This means spearheading change, but also living wellness personally within that change. Educational administration and policymakers do the same by championing well-being *as* curriculum. Every effort, at every level, creates more healthy thriving for all.

From the roots of safety, up the trunk of social well-being, and out through the branches of every domain, wellness is a diverse and collective journey. Students and teachers will improve their physical health, understand and appreciate emotions, flip negative thinking, discover meaning, or enjoy healthy relationships. Along the way, some might also find an ultimate purpose, or transcend separateness to realize that we are all made of love together. What makes any of this possible are teachers with the courage and imagination to live the questions of well-being with students, and create flourishing classrooms for a thriving world.

Closing Circle Activity (Main Move)

> "Step out of the circle of time and into the circle of love."
>
> —Rumi

As a classroom community matures through the exploration of well-being and learning, the potential for a deep and sacred closing circle experience grows. A circle held near the end of a group's time together reveals and celebrates connection, growth, and meaning. Knowing this circle adds the potential for a transcendent experience of appreciation and love. Teachers and students simultaneously feel regret and gratitude, knowing they will never be together in this same way again.

A closing circle can go in many directions, with the choice of circle prompts guided by the participants. No facilitator is needed, as teachers have learned to also be students of wellness, just as students have learned to be teachers, transcending their fixed roles. Prompts are in no particular order, and there is no requirement for everyone to respond. However the year has gone, a closing circle shows that the whole is not just greater than the sum of the parts, but that there truly are no parts in the first place.

Summary: Explore each well-being domain and say goodbye in a final classroom circle.
Time: 60 minutes
Trust Required: Medium

1. Prep (8 minutes): Print out the questions in table 11.1, along with any curriculum questions, inspiring quotations, or other prompts desired. Questions can also be added from particular domains of well-being. Make copies of this list and cut out each prompt on a separate slip so there are three or so copies of each. Spread these out randomly on windowsills and tables in the classroom. Gather any circle elements the class has adopted, such as a talking piece.
2. Gathering (2 minutes): Invite the class to circulate silently and read the various prompts, picking up one or two slips that resonate for them personally, and bring them back to sit silently in the circle when they are ready.
3. *Closing Circle* (45 minutes): When everyone is seated with their prompts, invite everyone to take refuge (p. 17) or use a mindful moment (p. 145). After this pause, prompts are read aloud to invite responses. New prompts will arise when the time is right for the first to end. Continue until everyone who wishes to share has done so.
4. *Last word* (5 minutes): Invite each student in a sequential round to speak a single word, whatever word summarizes their feelings or experience in the moment. Continue cycling around the circle with each participant saying a single word, even if it is the same word over and over. After a few rounds of this, invite students to take a final, silent reflection.
5. *Safety*: Final circles are for classes where relationships have gelled, and several domains of well-being have been explored. Ensure all students have had a chance to share by checking in with those who have not. Students may wish to just be there and listen.

6. *Integration Strategy*: Include prompts and questions related to overarching themes and major learning expectations in the curriculum, inviting reflection on program learning and well-being learning to blend.
7. *Schoolwide Extension*: Consider having such a circle with a committee, team, whole staff, or any group in the school. Closing in a good way acknowledges achievements made, growth realized, and love shared.

Table 11.1. Closing Circle Questions, Quotations and Prompts

"The beauty of the Circle is that we cannot see each other's back; and the strength of the Circle is that we can only see each other's beauty."

—Angaangaq Angakkorsuaq

Domain	Prompts (explore growth, changes, insights, and more)
Safety	My relationship with my personal needs, freedoms, and safety . . .
Cognitive	My relationship with my thoughts and cognitive well-being . . .
Emotional	My relationship with my feelings and emotional well-being . . .
Environmental	My relationship with the natural world and environmental well-being . . .
Eudaimonia	My relationship with what's most important to me, and about me . . .
Physical	My relationship with my body and physical well-being . . .
Resilience	My relationship with challenges and my capacity for resilience . . .
Social	My relationship with others and social well-being . . .
Spiritual	My relationship with my spirit and spiritual well-being . . .
Quotations	[Include a few quotations that resonate.]
Curriculum	[Include curricular reflection prompts as appropriate.]
Overall	What does well-being mean to you, compared to the start of this class?
Overall	An experience or relationship in this class I will remember . . .
Overall	My wish for everyone . . .

Keywords: caring, cognitive, circle, collaborative, choice, emotional, environmental, eudaimonia, foundational, hedonia, identity, integration, mindfulness, physical, resilience, safety, social, spiritual

APPENDIX A

Achievements Unlocked

Congratulations! By reaching this point, you have unlocked the achievements below. Completing them is up to you, as the eudaimonic reward is in the achieving itself.

Bronze

- ☐ *Well Met*: Use an activity personally before trying it with students in the classroom.
- ☐ *Toe in the Water*: Use any activity (or supplement) with students.
- ☐ *Share the Wealth*: Share your classroom well-being efforts with a colleague and a friend.
- ☐ *One Card Short*: Give away one card (see p. 263).

Silver

- ☐ *Moving Upstream*: Use any three activities (or supplements) with students.
- ☐ *Creativity is Joy*: Create your own wellness activity and use it with students.

- ☐ *Well Said*: Explain the nine domains of well-being to three other people.
- ☐ *Share the Wealth*: Give away four cards (one each to a student, colleague, friend, and relative)

Gold

- ☐ *Rainbow Unicorn*: Use at least one activity from each domain with students.
- ☐ *In Class We Trust*: Use three activities requiring high trust with students.
- ☐ *Well Versed*: Share well-being strategies with colleagues in a learning session or staff meeting.
- ☐ *Giving It All Away*: Give away this book in its entirety.

APPENDIX B

Activity Keywords

The keywords used throughout the book identify various characteristics of the activities that might be useful to educators seeking particular aspects.

- *card*—provided in brief on a shareable card (see p. 263 for cards)
- *caring*—supports caring for self or others
- *choice*—offers some degree of student voice/choice
- *circle*—conducted in a circle and develops circle-based capacity
- *cognitive*—cultivates cognitive well-being (domain)
- *collaborative*—requires groups to work together
- *creative*—develops imagination and originality
- *emotional*—cultivates emotional well-being (domain)
- *empower*—develops personal power or shares power
- *environmental*—cultivates environmental well-being (domain)
- *eudaimonia*—cultivates eudaimonic well-being (domain)
- *foundational*—usable in almost any context as a "main move"
- *get-to-know*—helps people learn more about each other in a group
- *gratitude*—develops gratitude
- *hedonia*—cultivates hedonic well-being: pleasure and satisfaction
- *icebreaker*—warm-up activity to begin things off, especially with new groups

- *identity*—explores aspects of self and personal identity
- *integration*—integrated into daily routines, teaching, learning, assessment, etc.
- *journal*—makes use of a self-reflective writing process or explicit journal entry
- *lifeplay*—invites usage and exploration throughout life beyond the classroom
- *mindfulness*—develops awareness, equanimity and other aspects of mindfulness
- *outdoor*—typically conducted in an outdoor setting
- *physical*—cultivates physical well-being (domain)
- *prep-free*—requires no material or prior preparation
- *resilience*—cultivates resilience (domain)
- *restorative*—repairs harm and restores relationships
- *safety*—preserves and cultivates safety (domain)
- *school-wide*—scalable for use across the school
- *short-'n'-safe*—takes less than five minutes and requires minimal classroom trust
- *social*—cultivates social well-being (domain)
- *space*—relates to the classroom's physical environment
- *spiritual*—cultivates spiritual well-being (domain)
- *support*—supports vulnerable students
- *time-maker*—potentially saves more time than it takes

APPENDIX C

Wellness is in the Cards

The cards in this section are designed to be shared with students, colleagues, parents, family, friends, community members, and others.[1] These summarized activities, selected from a variety of domains, are suitable for a range of ages and contexts beyond school. These cards can be cut from the book and given away, copied, or simply photographed and shared electronically.

---

1. Sharing of these pages is authorized for non-commercial, educational purposes.

TAKING REFUGE

1. Pick a haven that feels good:
   - listen to sounds
   - feel your body
   - notice your breathing
   - [create your own]

2. Remember three life cues:
   - an everyday thing (e.g., checking time)
   - a small challenge (e.g., traffic)
   - something planted (e.g., sticker on phone).

3. For two weeks, when you notice any cue (#2), take refuge (#1) for a moment, ten seconds, or more.

Scan here for more from the book *Flourishing Classrooms: A Deep Dive into Proactive Wellness for Grades 7–12*

TALK ABOUT ANYTHING

Ask these questions when something significant happens, and is calling to be explored in words.

1. What happened?
2. What were you thinking?
3. What were you feeling?
4. What was the impact?
5. Is there any meaning, growth, or connection to find in this?
6. What could change, in a good way?

Scan here for more from the book *Flourishing Classrooms: A Deep Dive into Proactive Wellness for Grades 7–12*

PARTNER LIFELINES

1. With a friend, take time to each draw a line representing your life.

2. Reflect silently on your own line, noting what stands out for you.

3. Share your lines and stories with each other as you wish, and anything you notice or feel.

4. Describe when your line changed, from up to down, or down to up.

5. What was bad about the up?
   What was good about the down?

Scan here for more from the book *Flourishing Classrooms: A Deep Dive into Proactive Wellness for Grades 7–12*

MINDFUL MOMENTS

1. Take five easy breaths, hands lovingly on the belly.

2. Trace each finger slowly, breathing up one side, down the other.

3. See anything fresh—with no intention of describing or judging it.

4. Do a routine task with absolute presence, immersing yourself.

5. When moving through any door, breathe, relax, and become aware.

Scan here for more from the book *Flourishing Classrooms: A Deep Dive into Proactive Wellness for Grades 7–12*

SELF-LOVE ACRONYM

1. Create a personal self-love acronym, such as:

   a. *SHAPED* by self-care = sleep, hike, authenticity, patience, express, drink water.

   b. Put on my *CAP* = calm, aware, presence.

   c. *REPEAT* daily = reps, exercise, protein, enjoy, asleep (by) ten.

2. When you remember the acronym, consider how you can love yourself.

Scan here for more from the book *Flourishing Classrooms: A Deep Dive into Proactive Wellness for Grades 7–12*

INTEROCEPTION: INQUIRING WITHIN

There are more than five senses, we can sense in as well as out, and interoception is feeling the body.

1. Sense the breath inside your body.

2. Where are emotions in your body, and what do they feel like?

3. *Inhabit* your head, then your heart, then gut, becoming each in turn.

4. Notice when something feels good/light/relaxed/warm inside versus bad/heavy/tight/cold.

Scan here for more from the book *Flourishing Classrooms: A Deep Dive into Proactive Wellness for Grades 7–12*

MINDFUL LISTENING

1. In any conversation, listen deeply.

   a. Make eye contact, put away technology, give yourself.

   b. Do not speak, or think of what you want to say.

   c. Listen with your body, mind, heart, and soul, and to what arises in you as you listen.

2. If the person pauses, listen. If they stop, ask "is there more?" and notice how the interaction deepens.

Scan here for more from the book *Flourishing Classrooms: A Deep Dive into Proactive Wellness for Grades 7–12*

WALK THE TALK

Try your next meeting (or friend chat) as a walking event rather than sitting. Move together in the same direction rather than sitting fixed opposite to one another.

1. Let people know ahead of time so they can dress accordingly.

2. Plan a quiet route near green space that allows side-by-side walking.

3. Groups of two to four are best.

4. Use phones to take notes, if needed.

Scan here for more from the book *Flourishing Classrooms: A Deep Dive into Proactive Wellness for Grades 7–12*

HEARTWARMING

Rub your hands softly to warm them.

1. Cup your hands on your cheeks to let warmth and gratitude flow to your creative, imaginative mind.

2. Cross your hands over your heart to let warmth and gratitude flow to your sensitive, feeling heart.

3. Place your hands on your belly to let warmth and gratitude flow to your marvelous, magnificent body.

4. Wrap your arms around yourself to embrace all of you.

Scan here for more from the book *Flourishing Classrooms: A Deep Dive into Proactive Wellness for Grades 7–12*

LOVING NOTES

Self-love is all-love: all ways, always.

1. Write a loving, self-compassionate text message to yourself at the beginning of each day, week, or season—as you feel it and need it.

2. Play your favorite love song, close your eyes, and *sing the words to yourself*, feeling the words are both *for* you and *from* you.

3. Write a love letter, on scented paper, and send it to yourself, along with a token of your deep self-affection.

Scan here for more from the book *Flourishing Classrooms: A Deep Dive into Proactive Wellness for Grades 7–12*

QUESTIONS OF PURPOSE

Marinate in these questions of meaning and share with those close to you.

1. What is your essential nature?
2. What is meaningful to you?
3. What do you get lost in?
4. What are your best qualities?
5. What do you like to work at?
6. What makes you feel alive?
7. What are you calling for, and what is the world calling of you?

Scan here for more from the book *Flourishing Classrooms: A Deep Dive into Proactive Wellness for Grades 7–12*

GRATITUDINALS

1. Play gratitude tennis with a friend, taking turns thinking of what you appreciate. Go for an epic rally.
2. Transform a thoughtless, oft-repeated act (like picking up your phone) into a moment to think of something you are grateful for.
3. Tell people, in person, out loud, what you appreciate about them.
4. Do a gratitude workout: three sets of 5-15 reps each of things, people, and situations you appreciate.

Scan here for more from the book *Flourishing Classrooms: A Deep Dive into Proactive Wellness for Grades 7–12*

SLEEP HYGIENE-O-METER

- Consistent wake-up and bed time.
- Comfortable bed and pillows.
- Bedroom cooler than 18°C or 67°F.
- Bedroom pitch black.
- Quiet area to sleep, no pet visits.
- Physically active during the day.
- No caffeine 6 hours before bed.
- No light/screens 2 hours before bed.
- Peaceful bedtime routine.
- Sleep aid such as a warm shower, print book, meditation, eye cover, ear plugs, white noise machine.

Week 1 _____/10   Week 2 _____/10   Week 3 _____/10

Scan here for more from the book *Flourishing Classrooms: A Deep Dive into Proactive Wellness for Grades 7–12*

N.E.A.T.

Non-exercise activity thermogenesis increases movement and boosts energy through non-exercise tasks.

1. Park as far as possible, rather than as close as possible.

2. Take the stairs.

3. Stand up to work on a computer.

4. Walk when on your phone.

5. _____

6. _____

Scan here for more from the book *Flourishing Classrooms: A Deep Dive into Proactive Wellness for Grades 7–12*

MINDFUL DIALOGUE

1. Person A shares for one minute, person B listens fully in silence.

2. Person B paraphrases back to person A what they heard and asks "Is that it?"

3. Person A confirms they got it (go to 4) or clarifies (back to 2).

4. Person B asks "Is there more?" (if yes, step 1, if no, step 5).

5. Switch roles, returning to step 1.

Scan here for more from the book *Flourishing Classrooms: A Deep Dive into Proactive Wellness for Grades 7–12*

F.A.R.M. THE JOY

Harvest good moments (sunsets, hugs) in your mind and heart long-term.

1. **F**ocus on the emotions, senses, and body feelings of the experience, completely immersing in it.

2. **A**ssociate the experience with other memories, noting what's new.

3. **R**emain in the experience for five, fifteen, thirty seconds or more.

4. **M**arinate in it all, letting it sink in and permeate your brain deeply.

Scan here for more from the book *Flourishing Classrooms: A Deep Dive into Proactive Wellness for Grades 7–12*

NOTES

PREFACE

1. Rainer Maria Rilke, and J. M. Burnham. "Letters to a Young Poet. 1934." Trans. MD Herter Norton. New York: WW Norton & Co (1993).

ACKNOWLEDGMENTS

1. Adams, Henry. *The Education of Henry Adams* (Franklin Library, 1983).

CHAPTER I

1. "Global Index: Overview." Social Progress Imperative, 2021. https://www.socialprogress.org/index/global.
2. "Home." Worldhappiness.report, March 31, 2021. https://worldhappiness.report/.
3. "The 17 Goals | Sustainable Development." UN.org, 2022. https://sdgs.un.org/goals.

4. OECD, PISA 2018 Results (Volume III): "What School Life Means for Students' Lives, 2019." (Paris: OECD Publishing). https://doi.org/10.1787/acd78851-en.

5. Moag-Stahlberg, Alicia, Nora Howley, and Lorry Luscri. "A National Snapshot of Local School Wellness Policies." *Journal of School Health* 78, no. 10 (2008): 562–68; Rosemarie O'Conner et al. "A Review of the Literature on Social and Emotional Learning for Students Ages 3–8." Regional Educational Laboratory Mid-Atlantic (2017); Zenner, Charlotte, Solveig Herrnleben-Kurz, and Harald Walach. "Mindfulness-Based Interventions in Schools—A Systematic Review and Meta-Analysis." *Frontiers in Psychology* 5 (2014): 603.

6. "Mathematics." Gov.on.ca, 2021. http://www.edu.gov.on.ca/eng/curriculum/secondary/curriculum-update.html.

7. Konu, Anne I., and Tomi P. Lintonen. "School Well-Being in Grades 4–12." *Health Education Research* 21, no. 5 (2006): 633–42.

8. Fowler, James H., and Nicholas A. Christakis. "Dynamic Spread of Happiness in a Large Social Network: Longitudinal Analysis over 20 Years in the Framingham Heart Study." *BMJ* 337 (2008).

9. Sacks, Vanessa, and David Murphey. "The Prevalence of Adverse Childhood Experiences, Nationally, by State, and by Race or Ethnicity," 2018.

10. Al Omari, Omar, Sulaiman Al Sabei, Omar Al Rawajfah, Loai Abu Sharour, Khalid Aljohani, Khaled Alomari, Lina Shkman, et al. "Prevalence and Predictors of Depression, Anxiety, and Stress among Youth at the Time of COVID-19: An Online Cross-Sectional Multicountry Study." Depression Research and Treatment 2020 (2020).

11. Xiang, Mi, Zhiruo Zhang, and Keisuke Kuwahara. "Impact of COVID-19 Pandemic on Children and Adolescents' Lifestyle Behavior Larger than Expected." *Progress in Cardiovascular Diseases* 63, no. 4 (July 2020): 531–32. https://doi.org/10.1016/j.pcad.2020.04.013.

12. Ghosh, Ritwik, Mahua J. Dubey, Subhankar Chatterjee, and Souvik Dubey. "Impact of COVID-19 on Children: Special Focus on the Psychosocial Aspect." *Minerva Pediatrica* 72, no. 3 (2020): 226–35.

13. Rozin, Paul, and Edward B. Royzman. "Negativity Bias, Negativity Dominance, and Contagion." *Personality and Social Psychology Review* 5, no. 4 (2001): 296–320.

14. Huppert, Felicia A., and Timothy T. C. So. "Flourishing across Europe: Application of a New Conceptual Framework for Defining Well-Being." *Social Indicators Research* 110, no. 3 (2013): 837–61.

15. Zola, Irving Kenneth. "The Problems and Prospects of Mutual Aid Groups." *Rehabilitation Psychology* 19, no. 4 (1972): 180.

16. Carr, Alan, Katie Cullen, Cora Keeney, Ciaran Canning, Olwyn Mooney, Ellen Chinseallaigh, and Annie O'Dowd. "Effectiveness of Positive Psychology Interventions: A Systematic Review and Meta-Analysis." *The Journal of Positive Psychology* 16, no. 6 (2021): 749–69.

17. Seligman, Martin E. P., and Mihaly Csikszentmihalyi. "Positive Psychology: An Introduction." In *Flow and the Foundations of Positive Psychology* (Springer, Dordrecht, 2014), 279–98.

18. Park, Nansook, Christopher Peterson, Daniel Szvarca, Randy J. Vander Molen, Eric S. Kim, and Kevin Collon. "Positive Psychology and Physical Health: Research and Applications." *American Journal of Lifestyle Medicine* 10, no. 3 (2016): 200–206.

19. Seligman, Martin E. P., *Learned Optimism: How to Change Your Mind and Your Life* (Vintage, 2006).

20. "The 10 Domains of Well-Being – Stanford BeWell." Stanford BeWell, April 24, 2017. https://bewell.stanford.edu/domains-well-being/.

21. Huppert and So. "Flourishing across Europe."

22. Seligman and Csikszentmihalyi. "Positive Psychology."

23. Ryff, Carol D. "Happiness Is Everything, or Is It? Explorations on the Meaning of Psychological Well-Being." *Journal of Personality and Social Psychology* 57, no. 6 (1989): 1069.

24. Keyes, Corey L. M. "The Mental Health Continuum: From Languishing to Flourishing in Life." *Journal of Health and Social Behavior* (2002): 207–22.

25. Gräbel, Bianca Friederike. "The Relationship between Wellbeing and Academic Achievement: A Systematic Review." Master's thesis, University of Twente, 2017.

26. Remen, Rachel Naomi. *My Grandfather's Blessings: Stories of Strength, Refuge, and Belonging* (Penguin, 2001).

27. White, Samantha. "Time to Think: Using Restorative Questions." International Institute for Restorative Practices. Retrieved from http://www.iirp.edu/news/1976-time-to-think-using-restorative-questions (2012).

28. Williams, Terry Tempest. *Refuge: An Unnatural History of Family and Place* (Vintage, 1992).

29. Small, Gary W., Jooyeon Lee, Aaron Kaufman, Jason Jalil, Prabha Siddarth, Himaja Gaddipati, Teena D. Moody, and Susan Y. Bookheimer. "Brain Health Consequences of Digital Technology Use." *Dialogues in Clinical Neuroscience* 22, no. 2 (2020): 179.

30. Ruiz, Don Miguel, and Janet Mills. *The Four Agreements (Illustrated Edition): A Practical Guide to Personal Freedom* (Four-Color Illustrated Ed.) (Hay House, Inc, 2011).

31. Soosalu, Grant, Suzanne Henwood, and Arun Deo. "Head, Heart, and Gut in Decision Making: Development of a Multiple Brain Preference Questionnaire." *SAGE Open* 9, no. 1 (2019): 2158244019837439.

32. Arnold, Andrew J., Piotr Winkielman, and Karen Dobkins. "Interoception and Social Connection." *Frontiers in Psychology* (2019): 2589.

33. Kanbara, Kenji, and Mikihiko Fukunaga. "Links among Emotional Awareness, Somatic Awareness and Autonomic Homeostatic Processing." *BioPsychoSocial Medicine* 10, no. 1 (2016): 1–11; Duschek, Stefan, Natalie S. Werner, Gustavo A. Reyes del Paso, and Rainer Schandry. "The Contributions of Interoceptive Awareness to Cognitive and Affective Facets of Body Experience. *Journal of Individual Differences* (2015).

34. Peterson, Christopher, and Martin E. P. Seligman. *Character Strengths and Virtues: A Handbook and Classification*. Vol. 1. (Oxford University Press, 2004).

35. Viacharacter.org. "Find Your 24 Character Strengths | Personal Strengths List | via Institute," 2019. https://www.viacharacter.org/character-strengths.

CHAPTER 2

1. Sacks, Vanessa, and David Murphey. "The Prevalence of Adverse Childhood Experiences, Nationally, by State, and by Race or Ethnicity." Dspacedirect.org, 2018.

2. Kendi, Ibram X. *How to Be an Antiracist* (One World, 2019).

3. Brown, Brené. *Braving the Wilderness: The Quest for True Belonging and the Courage to Stand Alone* (Random House, 2017).

4. Edutopia. "Daniel Goleman: The Emotional Atmosphere of a Classroom Matters." YouTube, October 8, 2013. https://youtu.be/MikBRguJq0g?t=38.

5. Cheryan, Sapna, Sianna A. Ziegler, Victoria C. Plaut, and Andrew N. Meltzoff. "Designing Classrooms to Maximize Student Achievement." *Policy Insights from the Behavioral and Brain Sciences* 1, no. 1 (2014): 4–12.

6. Barrett, Peter, Fay Davies, Yufan Zhang, and Lucinda Barrett. "The Impact of Classroom Design on Pupils' Learning: Final Results of a Holistic, Multi-Level Analysis." *Building and Environment* 89 (2015): 118–33.

7. Blair, Clancy, and Adele Diamond. "Biological Processes in Prevention and Intervention: The Promotion of Self-Regulation as a Means of Preventing School Failure." *Development and Psychopathology* 20, no. 3 (2008): 899–911.

8. Kohli, Rita, and Daniel G. Solórzano. "Teachers, Please Learn our Names!: Racial Microaggressions and the K–12 Classroom." *Race Ethnicity and Education* 15, no. 4 (2012): 441–62.

9. Roorda, Debora L., Helma M. Y. Koomen, Jantine L. Spilt, and Frans J. Oort. "The Influence of Affective Teacher–Student Relationships on Students' School Engagement and Achievement: A Meta-Analytic Approach." *Review of Educational Research* 81, no. 4 (2011): 493–529.

CHAPTER 3

1. The practice of savoring literally rewires your brain for wellness. For more self-directed neuroplasticity, see p. 156.
2. Herrmann, Esther, Josep Call, María Hernández-Lloreda, Brian Hare, and Michael Tomasello. "Humans Have Evolved Specialized Skills of Social Cognition: The Cultural Intelligence Hypothesis." *Science* 317, no. 5843 (2007).
3. Brown, Brené. *The Gifts of Imperfection* (Hazelden Publishing, 2010).
4. Berkman, Lisa F., and S. Leonard Syme. "Social Networks, Host Resistance, and Mortality: A Nine-Year Follow-Up Study of Alameda County Residents." *American Journal of Epidemiology* 109, no. 2 (1979): 186–204.
5. Stokes, Jeffrey E., and Sara M. Moorman. "Influence of the Social Network on Married and Unmarried Older Adults' Mental Health." *The Gerontologist* 58, no. 6 (2018): 1109–13.
6. Brannan, Debi, Robert Biswas-Diener, Cynthia D. Mohr, Shahrnaz Mortazavi, and Noah Stein. "Friends and Family: A Cross-Cultural Investigation of Social Support and Subjective Well-Being among College Students." *The Journal of Positive Psychology* 8, no. 1 (2013): 65–75.
7. Argyle, Michael. *The Psychology of Happiness* (Routledge, 2013).
8. Fowler, James H. "Dynamic Spread of Happiness in a Large Social Network: Longitudinal Analysis over 20 Years in the Framingham Heart Study." *BMJ* 337, no. a2338: 1–9. doi:https://doi.org/10.1136/bmj.a2338.
9. Gallagher, Emily. "The Effects of Teacher-Student Relationships: Social and Academic Outcomes of Low-Income Middle and High School Students" (2019). https://wp.nyu.edu/steinhardt-appsych_opus/the-effects-of-teacher-student-relationships-social-and-academic-outcomes-of-low-income-middle-and-high-school-students/.
10. Norman-Murch, Trudi. "Keeping Our Balance on a Slippery Slope: Training and Supporting Infant/Family Specialists within an Organizational Context." *Infants & Young Children* 18, no. 4 (2005): 308–22.
11. "Social-Emotional Learning (SEL) Standards in All 50 States." Positive action.net, 2020. https://www.positiveaction.net/blog/sel-standards.
12. Garnett, Bernice Raveche, Colby T. Kervick, Mika Moore, Tracy A. Ballysingh, and Lance C. Smith. "School Staff and Youth Perspectives of Tier

1 Restorative Practices Classroom Circles." *School Psychology Review* (2020): 1–15; Augustine, C. H., J. Engberg, G. E. Grimm, E. Lee, E. L. Wang, K. Christianson, and A. A. Joseph. "Restorative Practices Help Reduce Student Suspensions" (2018).

13. Hess, Ursula. "Who to Whom and Why: The Social Nature of Emotional Mimicry." *Psychophysiology* 58, no. 1 (2021): e13675; Walter, Henrik. "Social Cognitive Neuroscience of Empathy: Concepts, Circuits, and Genes." *Emotion Review* 4, no. 1 (2012): 9–17.

14. Arslan, Gökmen. "Understanding the Association between School Belonging and Emotional Health in Adolescents." *International Journal of Educational Psychology* 7, no. 1 (2018): 21–41; Allen, Kelly-Ann, Christopher D. Slaten, Gökmen Arslan, Sue Roffey, Heather Craig, and Dianne A. Vella-Brodrick. "School Belonging: The Importance of Student and Teacher Relationships." In *The Palgrave Handbook of Positive Education*, Margaret L. Kern and Michael L. Wehmeyer (Eds.) (Palgrave Macmillan, Cham, 2021), 525–50; Tillery, Amy Dutton, Kris Varjas, Andrew T. Roach, Gabriel P. Kuperminc, and Joel Meyers. "The Importance of Adult Connections in Adolescents' Sense of School Belonging: Implications for Schools and Practitioners." *Journal of School Violence* 12, no. 2 (2013): 134–55.

15. Merton, Thomas. *Conjectures of a Guilty Bystander* (Doubleday, 1966).

16. Algoe, Sara B., and Jonathan Haidt. "Witnessing Excellence in Action: The 'Other-Praising' Emotions of Elevation, Gratitude, and Admiration." *The Journal of Positive Psychology* 4, no. 2 (2009): 105–27.

17. Pohling, Rico, and Rhett Diessner. "Moral Elevation and Moral Beauty: A Review of the Empirical Literature." *Review of General Psychology* 20, no. 4 (2016): 412–25.

18. Gillham, Jane, Zoe Adams-Deutsch, Jaclyn Werner, Karen Reivich, Virginia Coulter-Heindl, Mark Linkins, Breanna Winder, et al. "Character Strengths Predict Subjective Well-Being during Adolescence." *The Journal of Positive Psychology* 6, no. 1 (2011): 31–44.

19. Cook, Clayton R., Aria Fiat, Madeline Larson, Christopher Daikos, Tal Slemrod, Elizabeth A. Holland, Andrew J. Thayer, and Tyler Renshaw. "Positive Greetings at the Door: Evaluation of a Low-Cost, High-Yield Proactive Classroom Management Strategy." *Journal of Positive Behavior Interventions* 20, no. 3 (2018): 149–59.

20. Allday, R. Allan, and Kerri Pakurar. "Effects of Teacher Greetings on Student On-Task Behavior." *Journal of Applied Behavior Analysis* 40, no. 2 (2007): 317–20.

21. Fipps, Lisa. *Starfish* (Nancy Paulsen Books, 2021).

22. Metatawabin, Edmund, and Alexandra Shimo. *Up Ghost River: A Chief's Journey through the Turbulent Waters of Native History* (Vintage Canada, 2015).

23. Quoted with permission of Jack Kornfield. "Seeing the Goodness in Another Being." YouTube Video. May 24, 2019. https://www.youtube.com/watch?v=0F2CF4Jc2mg&ab_channel=JackKornfield.

24. Ballard, Jamie. "During COVID, Many Millennials Still Feel Lonely." Yougov.com. YouGov, May 2020. https://today.yougov.com/topics/lifestyle/articles-reports/2020/05/01/loneliness-mental-health-coronavirus-poll-data.

25. Hunt, Melissa G., Rachel Marx, Courtney Lipson, and Jordyn Young. "No More FOMO: Limiting Social Media Decreases Loneliness and Depression." *Journal of Social and Clinical Psychology* 37, no. 10 (2018): 751–68.

26. Liljedahl, Peter. "The Affordances of Using Visibly Random Groups in a Mathematics Classroom." In *Transforming Mathematics Instruction* (Springer, Cham, 2014), pp. 127–44.

CHAPTER 4

1. Le Guin, Ursula K. *The Lathe of Heaven: A Novel* (Simon and Schuster, 2008).

2. Ekins, Emily E. "What Americans Think about Poverty, Wealth, and Work." The Cato Institute, September 24, 2019.

3. Lifeway Research. "Americans' Views of Life's Meaning and Purpose Are Changing—Lifeway Research," April 6, 2021. https://research.lifeway.com/2021/04/06/americans-views-of-lifes-meaning-and-purpose-are-changing/.

4. OECD, PISA 2018 Results (Volume III): *What School Life Means for Students' Lives, 2019*, OECD Publishing, Paris, https://doi.org/10.1787/acd78851-en.

5. Gentzler, Amy L., Katy L. DeLong, Cara A. Palmer, and Veronika Huta. "Hedonic and Eudaimonic Motives to Pursue Well-Being in Three Samples of Youth." *Motivation and Emotion* 45, no. 3 (2021): 312–26.

6. Huta, Veronika, and Alan S. Waterman. "Eudaimonia and Its Distinction from Hedonia: Developing a Classification and Terminology for Understanding Conceptual and Operational Definitions." *Journal of Happiness Studies* 15, no. 6 (2014): 1425–56.

7. Steger, Michael F. "Meaning and Well-Being." In *Handbook of Well-Being*, edited by E. Diener, S. Oishi, and L. Tay (DEF Publishers, 2018).

8. Schnell, Tatjana. "Individual Differences in Meaning-Making: Considering the Variety of Sources of Meaning, Their Density and Diversity." *Personality and Individual Differences* 51, no. 5 (2011): 667–73.

9. Schnell, Tatjana. "The Sources of Meaning and Meaning in Life Questionnaire (SoMe): Relations to Demographics and Well-Being." *The Journal of Positive Psychology* 4, no. 6 (2009): 483–99.

10. Frankl, Viktor E. *Man's Search for Meaning* (Simon and Schuster, 1985).

11. Diener, Ed, Richard E. Lucas, and Christie Napa Scollon. "Beyond the Hedonic Treadmill: Revising the Adaptation Theory of Well-Being." In *The Science of Well-Being* (Springer, Dordrecht, 2009), 103–118.

12. Gay, Roxane. "On Making Black Lives Matter." *Marie Claire*, July 11, 2016. https://www.marieclaire.com/culture/a21423/roxane-gay-philando-castile-alton-sterling/.

13. Marshall, Sheila K. "Do I Matter? Construct Validation of Adolescents' Perceived Mattering to Parents and Friends." *Journal of Adolescence* 24, no. 4 (2001): 473–90.

14. Fredrickson, Barbara. *Positivity: Groundbreaking Research to Release Your Inner Optimist and Thrive* (Simon and Schuster, 2010).

15. Steger, Michael F., Todd B. Kashdan, and Shigehiro Oishi. "Being Good by Doing Good: Daily Eudaimonic Activity and Well-Being." *Journal of Research in Personality* 42, no. 1 (2008): 22-42.

16. Steger et al., "Being Good by Doing Good."

17. Roberts, Laura Morgan, Jane E. Dutton, Gretchen M. Spreitzer, Emily D. Heaphy, and Robert E. Quinn. "Composing the Reflected Best-Self Portrait: Building Pathways for Becoming Extraordinary in Work Organizations." *Academy of Management Review* 30, no. 4 (2005): 712–36.

18. Hart, Roger A. "Children's Participation: From Tokenism to Citizenship." *Innocenti Essay* no. 4, 1992.

19. Morethanonestory.org. "More Than One Story," 2022. https://www.morethanonestory.org/en.

CHAPTER 5

1. Csikszentmihalyi, Mihaly. *Flow: The Classic Work on How to Achieve Happiness* (Random House, 2002).

2. Jennings, Herbert Spencer. *Behavior of the Lower Organisms*. No. 10 (Columbia University Press, 1906).

3. Reynierse, James H., and Gary L. Walsh. "Behavior Modification in the Protozoan Stentor Re-Examined." *The Psychological Record* 17, no. 2 (1967):

161–65; Dexter, Joseph P., Sudhakaran Prabakaran, and Jeremy Gunawardena. "A Complex Hierarchy of Avoidance Behaviors in a Single-Cell Eukaryote." *Current Biology* 29, no. 24 (2019): 4323–29.

4. Di Fabio, Annamaria, and Letizia Palazzeschi. "Hedonic and Eudaimonic Well-Being: The Role of Resilience beyond Fluid Intelligence and Personality Traits." *Frontiers in Psychology* 6 (2015): 1367.

5. Gillham, Jane, Rachel M. Abenavoli, Steven M. Brunwasser, Mark Linkins, Karen J. Reivich, and Martin E. P. Seligman. "Resilience Education" (2013).

6. Strauss, Valerie. "The Problem with Teaching "Grit" to Poor Kids? They Already Have It. Here's What They Really Need." *The Washington Post*, May 10, 2016, pp. 2016–18. https://www.washingtonpost.com/news/answer-sheet/wp/2016/05/10/the-problem-with-teaching-grit-to-poor-kids-they-already-have-it-heres-what-they-really-need/.

7. hooks, bell. *Feminist Theory: From Margin to Center* (Pluto Press, 2000).

8. Kim-Cohen, Julia. "Resilience and Developmental Psychopathology." *Child and Adolescent Psychiatric Clinics of North America* 16, no. 2 (2007): 271–83.

9. McLaren, Karla. *The Language of Emotions: What Your Feelings Are Trying to Tell You* (Sounds True, 2010).

10. Graham, Linda. Resilience: *Powerful Practices for Bouncing Back from Disappointment, Difficulty, and Even Disaster* (New World Library, 2018).

11. Reducing Overwhelm with the STOP Technique. https://thewellnesssociety.org/wp-content/uploads/2019/02/STOP-Technique-PDF-1.pdf.

12. Michele McDonald, "R.A.I.N. ~ D.R.O.P," Vipassana Hawai'i, August 28, 2020. https://vipassanahawaii.org/resources/raindrop/.

13. Tara Brach, "RAIN: A Practice of Radical Compassion," Published 2020. https://www.tarabrach.com/rain-practice-radical-compassion/.

14. Art Lockhart, "Forging Individual Transformation," *Gatehouse Adult Support Program Phase 2 Participant Manual*, http://thegatehouse.org/wp-content/uploads/2017/08/PH2-MANUAL-FINAL.pdf.

15. Ciolek, Joanna. "How to Release Emotions Stuck in Your Body." PACEsConnection, November 16, 2018. https://www.pacesconnection.com/blog/how-to-release-emotions-stuck-in-your-body.

16. Search Inside Yourself Leadership Institute. SIYLI. Published 2012. https://siyli.org/resources/mindfulness-and-negative-emotions.

17. *Oxford Dictionary of Proverbs* (Sixth edition). Edited by Jennifer Speake, Entry: "When one door shuts, another opens" (Oxford University Press, 2015). Accessed via Oxford Reference Online.

18. Tedeschi, Richard G., and Lawrence G. Calhoun. "Posttraumatic Growth: Conceptual Foundations and Empirical Evidence." *Psychological Inquiry* 15, no. 1 (2004): 1–18.

19. Having taught physics and mathematics for many years, I can say the answer is "too many."

20. Angelou, Maya. "Letter to My Daughter." GagasMedia, 2012.

21. Wachtel, Ted. "Restorative Justice Typology." 2016 International Institute for Restorative Practices. https://www.iirp.edu/defining-restorative/restorative-justice-typology

22. White, Samantha. "Time to Think: Using Restorative Questions." International Institute for Restorative Practices. Retrieved from https://www.iirp.edu/news/time-to-think-using-restorative-questions (2012).

23. IIRP. "What Is Restorative Practices?" https://www.iirp.edu/restorative-practices/what-is-restorative-practices.

24. Rick Hanson, "Hug the Monkey," May 26, 2020. https://www.rickhanson.net/hug-the-monkey/.

25. Dweck, Carol S. *Mindset: The New Psychology of Success*. (Random house, 2006).

CHAPTER 6

1. Foshay, Arthur W. "The Curriculum Matrix: Transcendence and Mathematics." *Journal of Curriculum and Supervision* 6, no. 4 (1991): 277–93.

2. Coker, David. "A Mission Statement Does Not a Mission Make: A Mixed Methods Investigation in Public Education." *International Education Studies* 15, no. 1 (2022): 210–25.

3. Schafft, Kai A., and Catharine Biddle. "Place and Purpose in Public Education: School District Mission Statements and Educational (Dis) Embeddedness." *American Journal of Education* 120, no. 1 (2013): 055–076.

4. Verger, Antoni, Lluís Parcerisa, and Clara Fontdevila. "The Growth and Spread of Large-Scale Assessments and Test-Based Accountabilities: A Political Sociology of Global Education Reforms." *Educational Review* 71, no. 1 (2019): 5–30.

5. "The Programme for International Student, Country Note, United States," 2019, https://www.oecd.org/pisa/publications/PISA2018_CN_USA.pdf.

6. Soosalu, Grant, Suzanne Henwood, and Arun Deo. "Head, Heart, and Gut in Decision Making: Development of a Multiple Brain Preference Questionnaire." *Sage Open* 9, no. 1 (2019): 2158244019837439; WELL For Life.

"Stanford WELL for Life," 2020. https://med.stanford.edu/wellforlife/research/stanford-well-for-life.html.

7. Pietarinen, Janne, Tiina Soini, and Kirsi Pyhältö. "Students' Emotional and Cognitive Engagement as the Determinants of Well-Being and Achievement in School." *International Journal of Educational Research* 67 (2014): 40–51.

8. Hanh, Thich Nhat. *The Miracle of Mindfulness, Gift Edition: An Introduction to the Practice of Meditation* (Beacon Press, 2016).

9. McKeering, Phillipa, and Yoon-Suk Hwang. "A Systematic Review of Mindfulness-Based School Interventions with Early Adolescents." *Mindfulness* 10, no. 4 (2019): 593–610; Zenner, Charlotte, Solveig Herrnleben-Kurz, and Harald Walach. "Mindfulness-Based Interventions in Schools—A Systematic Review and Meta-Analysis." *Frontiers in Psychology* 5 (2014): 603.

10. Wang, Claudia, Kaigang Li, and Susan Gaylord. "Prevalence, Patterns, and Predictors of Meditation Use among U.S. Children: Results from the National Health Interview Survey." *Complementary Therapies in Medicine* 43 (2019): 271–76.

11. Howarth, Ana, Jared G. Smith, Linda Perkins-Porras, and Michael Ussher. "Effects of Brief Mindfulness-Based Interventions on Health-Related Outcomes: A Systematic Review." *Mindfulness* 10, no. 10 (2019): 1957–68.

12. Schwartz, Jeffrey, and Sharon Begley. *The Mind and the Brain: Neuroplasticity and the Power of Mental Force* (Harper Collins, 2007).

13. Jose, Paul E., Bee T. Lim, and Fred B. Bryant. "Does Savoring Increase Happiness? A Daily Diary Study." *The Journal of Positive Psychology* 7, no. 3 (2012): 176–87; Klein, Tim, Beth Kendall, and Theresa Tougas. "Changing Brains, Changing Lives: Researching the Lived Experience of Individuals Practicing Self-Directed Neuroplasticity" (2019). Retrieved from Sophia, the St. Catherine University repository website: https://sophia.stkate.edu/ma_hhs/20.

14. Hanson, Rick, Shauna Shapiro, Emma Hutton-Thamm, Michael R. Hagerty, and Kevin P. Sullivan. "Learning to Learn from Positive Experiences." *The Journal of Positive Psychology* (2021): 1–12.

15. Larsen, Randy J., and Zvjezdana Prizmic. "Regulation of Emotional Well-Being: Overcoming the Hedonic Treadmill." In M. Eid and R. J. Larsen (Eds.), *The Science of Subjective Well-Being* (Guilford Press, 2008), 258–89.

16. Gable, Shelly L., Harry T. Reis, Emily A. Impett, and Evan R. Asher. "What Do You Do When Things Go Right? The Intrapersonal and Interpersonal Benefits of Sharing Positive Events." *Journal of Personality and Social Psychology* 87, no. 2 (2004): 228.

17. "Brain CORE" is one way to remember these steps. Another mnemonic is to "RECUPERATE mentally," also encapsulating the steps (reCUpErate, recUPERATE, REcuPErATe) with *uperate* as a play on operate, tilted upward.

18. Hanson, Rick, Shauna Shapiro, Emma Hutton-Thamm, Michael R. Hagerty, and Kevin P. Sullivan. "Learning to Learn from Positive Experiences." *The Journal of Positive Psychology* (2021): 1–12.

19. Csikszentmihalyi, Mihaly. *Flow: The Psychology of Optimal Experience* (New York: Harper & Row, 1990).

20. Michailidis, Lazaros, Emili Balaguer-Ballester, and Xun He. "Flow and Immersion in Video Games: The Aftermath of a Conceptual Challenge." *Frontiers in Psychology* 9 (2018): 1682.

21. Csikszentmihalhi, Mihaly. *Finding Flow: The Psychology of Engagement with Everyday Life* (Hachette UK, 2020).

22. Csikszentmihalyi, Mihaly, Sami Abuhamdeh, and Jeanne Nakamura. "Flow." In *Flow and the Foundations of Positive Psychology* (Springer, Dordrecht, 2014), 227–38.

23. Terada, Youki. "Research-Tested Benefits of Breaks." Edutopia. George Lucas Educational Foundation, March 9, 2018. https://www.edutopia.org/article/research-tested-benefits-breaks.

24. Mantzios, Michail, and Kyriaki Giannou. "When Did Coloring Books Become Mindful? Exploring the Effectiveness of a Novel Method of Mindfulness-Guided Instructions for Coloring Books to Increase Mindfulness and Decrease Anxiety." *Frontiers in Psychology* 9 (2018): 56.

25. Boller, Barbara. "Teaching Organizational Skills in Middle School: Moving toward Independence." *The Clearing House: A Journal of Educational Strategies, Issues and Ideas* 81, no. 4 (2008): 169–71

CHAPTER 7

1. McLaren, Karla. *The Language of Emotions: What Your Feelings Are Trying to Tell You* (Sounds True, 2010).

2. Amedie, Jacob. "The Impact of Social Media on Society." (2015). *Pop Culture Intersections*. 2. https://scholarcommons.scu.edu/engl_176/2.

3. Google Trends, 2015. https://trends.google.com/trends/explore?date=all&q=social%20emotional%20learning.

4. Dermody, C., and L. Dusenbury. (2022) 2022 *Social and Emotional Learning State Scorecard Scan* (Chicago: Collaborative for Academic, Social and Emotional Learning).

5. "Human Abilities: Emotional Intelligence." *Annual Reviews*, 2015; Durlak, Joseph A., Roger P. Weissberg, Allison B. Dymnicki, Rebecca D. Taylor,

and Kriston B. Schellinger. "The Impact of Enhancing Students' Social and Emotional Learning: A Meta-Analysis of School-Based Universal Interventions." *Child Development* 82, no. 1 (2011): 405–32.

6. Seligman, M. E. P., and A. Adler. (2018). "Positive Education." *Global Happiness Policy Report*, 52–73. https://s3.amazonaws.com/ghc-2018/GHC_Ch4.pdf.

7. Lyubomirsky, Sonja, Kennon M. Sheldon, and David Schkade. "Pursuing Happiness: The Architecture of Sustainable Change." *Review of General Psychology* 9, no. 2 (2005): 111–31.

8. Kotsou, Ilios, Moira Mikolajczak, Alexandre Heeren, Jacques Grégoire, and Christophe Leys. "Improving Emotional Intelligence: A Systematic Review of Existing Work and Future Challenges." *Emotion Review* 11, no. 2 (2019): 151–65.

9. Plutchik, Robert. *The Emotions* (University Press of America, 1991), 111.

10. Cowen, Alan S., Dacher Keltner, Florian Schroff, Brendan Jou, Hartwig Adam, and Gautam Prasad. "Sixteen Facial Expressions Occur in Similar Contexts Worldwide." *Nature* 589, no. 7841 (2021): 251–57.

11. Côté, Stéphane, Anett Gyurak, and Robert W. Levenson. "The Ability to Regulate Emotion Is Associated with Greater Well-Being, Income, and Socioeconomic Status." *Emotion* 10, no. 6 (2010): 923.

12. Campbell-Sills, Laura, David H. Barlow, Timothy A. Brown, and Stefan G. Hofmann. "Effects of Suppression and Acceptance on Emotional Responses of Individuals with Anxiety and Mood Disorders." *Behaviour Research and Therapy* 44, no. 9 (2006): 1251–63.; Srivastava, Sanjay, Maya Tamir, Kelly M. McGonigal, Oliver P. John, and James J. Gross. "The Social Costs of Emotional Suppression: A Prospective Study of the Transition to College." *Journal of Personality and Social Psychology* 96, no. 4 (2009): 883.

13. McLaren, Karla. *The Language of Emotions: What Your Feelings Are Trying to Tell You* (Sounds True, 2010).

14. McGonigal, Kelly. *How to Make Stress Your Friend*. Ted Global, Edinburgh, Scotland 6 (2013): 13. https://www.youtube.com/watch?v=RcGyVTAoXEU.

15. Cooper, Damian. *Rebooting Assessment: A Practical Guide for Balancing Conversations, Performances, and Products* (Solution Tree Press, 2022).

16. Stamen Design. *The Ekmans' Atlas of Emotion*. 2022. http://atlasofemotions.org/.

17. Wood, Alex M., Jeffrey J. Froh, and Adam W. A. Geraghty. "Gratitude and Well-Being: A Review and Theoretical Integration." *Clinical Psychology Review* 30, no. 7 (2010): 890–905.

18. Bluth, Karen, and Kristin D. Neff. "New Frontiers in Understanding the Benefits of Self-Compassion." *Self and Identity* 17, no. 6 (2018): 605–8.

CHAPTER 8

1. Macy, Joanna. *World as Lover, World as Self: Courage for Global Justice and Planetary Renewal* (Parallax Press, 2021).
2. Saunders, Travis J., and Jeff K. Vallance. "Screen Time and Health Indicators among Children and Youth: Current Evidence, Limitations and Future Directions." *Applied Health Economics and Health Policy* 15, no. 3 (2017): 323–31.
3. Pritchard, Alison, Miles Richardson, David Sheffield, and Kirsten McEwan. "The Relationship between Nature Connectedness and Eudaimonic Well-Being: A Meta-Analysis." *Journal of Happiness Studies* 21, no. 3 (2020): 1145–67.
4. Nisbet, Elizabeth, John Zelenski, and Steven Murphy. "The Nature Relatedness Scale: Linking Individuals' Connection with Nature to Environmental Concern." *Environment and Behavior* 41, no. 5 (2009): 715–40.
5. Howell, Andrew J., Raelyne L. Dopko, Holli-Anne Passmore, and Karen Buro. "Nature Connectedness: Associations with Well-Being and Mindfulness." *Personality and Individual Differences* 51, no. 2 (2011): 166–71.
6. Nisbet, Elizabeth K., John M. Zelenski, and Steven A. Murphy. "Happiness Is in Our Nature: Exploring Nature Relatedness as a Contributor to Subjective Well-Being." *Journal of Happiness Studies* 12, no. 2 (2011): 303–22.
7. Ryan, Richard M., Netta Weinstein, Jessey Bernstein, Kirk Warren Brown, Louis Mistretta, and Marylene Gagne. "Vitalizing Effects of Being Outdoors and in Nature." *Journal of Environmental Psychology* 30, no. 2 (2010): 159–68.
8. Taylor, Steve, and Krisztina Egeto-Szabo. "Exploring Awakening Experiences: A Study of Awakening Experiences in Terms of Their Triggers, Characteristics, Duration and After Effects." *Journal of Transpersonal Psychology* 49, no. 1 (2017): 45–65.
9. Nature Relatedness. "What Is Nature Relatedness? | Nature Relatedness," 2015. https://www.naturerelatedness.ca/what-is-nature-relatedness.
10. O'Brien, Liz. "Learning Outdoors: The Forest School Approach." *Education 3–13*, 37, no. 1 (2009): 45–60.
11. Waite, Sue, Rowena Passy, Martin Gilchrist, Anne Hunt, and Ian Blackwell. "Natural Connections Demonstration Project, 2012–2016." *Natural Connections Demonstration Project, 2012–2016: Final Report* (2016).
12. Ajiboye, Josiah O., and Sunday Adekojo Olatundun. "Impact of Some Environmental Education Outdoor Activities on Nigerian Primary School Pupils' Environmental Knowledge." *Applied Environmental Education and Communication* 9, no. 3 (2010): 149–58.

13. Damen, Ida, Carine Lallemand, Rens Brankaert, Aarnout Brombacher, Pieter Van Wesemael, and Steven Vos. "Understanding Walking Meetings: Drivers and Barriers." In *Proceedings of the 2020 CHI Conference on Human Factors in Computing Systems* (2020), pp. 1–14.

14. Economy, Peter. "7 Powerful Reasons to Take Your Next Meeting for a Walk." Inc.com. *Inc.*, April 6, 2015. https://www.inc.com/peter-economy/7-powerful-reasons-to-take-your-next-meeting-for-a-walk.html; Oppezzo, Marily, and Daniel L. Schwartz. "Give Your Ideas Some Legs: The Positive Effect of Walking on Creative Thinking." *Journal of Experimental Psychology: Learning, Memory, and Cognition* 40, no. 4 (2014): 1142–52. https://doi.org/10.1037/a0036577.

15. Louv, Richard. *Last Child in the Woods: Saving Our Children from Nature-Deficit Disorder* (Algonquin Books, 2008).

16. Benfield, Jacob A., Gretchen Nurse Rainbolt, Paul A. Bell, and Geoffrey H. Donovan. "Classrooms with Nature Views: Evidence of Differing Student Perceptions and Behaviors." *Environment and Behavior* 47, no. 2 (2015):140–57.

17. UN.org. "Eco-Green Clubs in Schools—United Nations Partnerships for SDGs Platform," 2021. https://sdgs.un.org/partnerships/eco-green-clubs-schools.

CHAPTER 9

1. World Health Organization. "Constitution of the World Health Organization," 2022. https://www.who.int/about/governance/constitution.

2. Guthold, Regina, Gretchen A. Stevens, Leanne M. Riley, and Fiona C. Bull. "Global Trends in Insufficient Physical Activity among Adolescents: A Pooled Analysis of 298 Population-Based Surveys with 1.6 Million Participants." *The Lancet Child & Adolescent Health* 4, no. 1 (2020): 23–35.

3. Wheaton, Anne G., Sherry Everett Jones, Adina C. Cooper, and Janet B. Croft. "Short Sleep Duration among Middle School and High School Students—United States, 2015." *Morbidity and Mortality Weekly Report* 67, no. 3 (2018): 85.

4. Liu, Junxiu, Colin D. Rehm, Jennifer Onopa, and Dariush Mozaffarian. "Trends in Diet Quality among Youth in the United States, 1999–2016." *Journal of the American Medical Association* 323, no. 12 (2020): 1161–74.

5. Kearney-Cooke, Ann, and Diana Tieger. "Development of Eating Disorders." In *The Wiley Handbook of Eating Disorders*, edited by Linda Smolak and Michael P. Levine (Wiley-Blackwell, 2015): 285.

6. Aronson, Elliot, and Diane Bridgeman. "Jigsaw Groups and the Desegregated Classroom: In Pursuit of Common Goals." *Personality and Social Psychology Bulletin* 5, no. 4 (1979): 438–46.

7. Gallant, Janae, and Megan Lamb. "Health at Every Size (HAES)—What's It All About? – Obesity Canada." Obesity Canada, April 6, 2018. https://obesitycanada.ca/snp/health-at-every-size-haes-whats-it-all-about/.

8. Donskoy, Innessa, and Darius Loghmanee. "Insomnia in Adolescence." *Medical Sciences* 6, no. 3 (2018): 72.

9. Nedeltcheva, Arlet V., Jennifer M. Kilkus, Jacqueline Imperial, Dale A. Schoeller, and Plamen D. Penev. "Insufficient Sleep Undermines Dietary Efforts to Reduce Adiposity." *Annals of Internal Medicine* 153, no. 7 (2010): 435–41; Dolezal, Brett A., Eric V. Neufeld, David M. Boland, Jennifer L. Martin, and Christopher B. Cooper. "Interrelationship between Sleep and Exercise: A Systematic Review." *Advances in Preventive Medicine* (2017).

10. Amschler, Denise H., and James F. McKenzie. "Perceived Sleepiness, Sleep Habits and Sleep Concerns of Public School Teachers, Administrators and Other Personnel." *American Journal of Health Education* 41, no. 2 (2010): 102–9.

11. Levine, James A., Mark W. Vander Weg, James O. Hill, and Robert C. Klesges. "Non-exercise Activity Thermogenesis: The Crouching Tiger Hidden Dragon of Societal Weight Gain." *Arteriosclerosis, Thrombosis, and Vascular Biology* 26, no. 4 (2006): 729–36.

12. Danquah, Ida H., and Janne S. Tolstrup. "Standing Meetings Are Feasible and Effective in Reducing Sitting Time among Office Workers—Walking Meetings Are Not: Mixed-Methods Results on the Feasibility and Effectiveness of Active Meetings Based on Data from the 'Take a Stand!' Study." *International Journal of Environmental Research and Public Health* 17, no. 5 (March 5, 2020): 1713. https://doi.org/10.3390/ijerph17051713.

13. Bluedorn, Allen C., Daniel B. Turban, and Mary Sue Love. "The Effects of Stand-Up and Sit-Down Meeting Formats on Meeting Outcomes." *Journal of Applied Psychology* 84, no. 2 (1999): 277.

CHAPTER 10

1. Kessler, Rachael. *The Soul of Education: Helping Students Find Connection, Compassion, and Character at School* (Association for Supervision and Curriculum Development, 2000).

2. Gomez, Rapson, and John W. Fisher. "Domains of Spiritual Well-Being and Development and Validation of the Spiritual Well-Being Questionnaire."

Personality and Individual Differences 35, no. 8 (2003): 1975–1991; Vimal, Rām Lakhan Pāndey. "Meanings Attributed to the Term 'Spirituality' and Science Underlying It." *Vision Research Institute: Living Vision and Consciousness Research* 7, no. 5 (2015): 1–30.

3. Worldpopulationreview.com. "Religion by Country 2022," 2022. https://worldpopulationreview.com/country-rankings/religion-by-country.

4. Benson, Peter L., Peter C. Scales, Amy K. Syvertsen, and Eugene C. Roehlkepartain. "Is Youth Spiritual Development a Universal Developmental Process? An International Exploration." *The Journal of Positive Psychology* 7, no. 6 (2012): 453–70.

5. United Nations. "Universal Declaration of Human Rights, Article 18." UN General Assembly 302, no. 2 (1948).

6. Taylor, Steve, and Krisztina Egeto-Szabo. "Exploring Awakening Experiences: A Study of Awakening Experiences in Terms of Their Triggers, Characteristics, Duration and After Effects." *Journal of Transpersonal Psychology* 49, no. 1 (2017).

7. Preston, Jesse L., and Faith Shin. "Spiritual Experiences Evoke Awe through the Small Self in Both Religious and Non-Religious Individuals." *Journal of Experimental Social Psychology* 70 (2017): 212–21.

8. Michaelson, Valerie, Nathan King, Jo Inchley, Dorothy Currie, Fiona Brooks, and William Pickett. "Domains of Spirituality and Their Associations with Positive Mental Health: A Study of Adolescents in Canada, England and Scotland." *Preventive Medicine* 125 (2019): 12–18.

9. Keltner, Dacher, and Jonathan Haidt. "Approaching Awe, a Moral, Spiritual, and Aesthetic Emotion." *Cognition and Emotion* 17, no. 2 (2003): 297–314.

10. Marcus Aurelius, Emperor of Rome, 121–180. *The Meditations of Marcus Aurelius* (Peter Pauper Press, 1942).

11. Ray, Amit. *Meditation: Insights and Inspirations* (Inner Life Publishers, 2010).

12. Duerr, M. *A Powerful Silence: The Role of Meditation and Other Contemplative Practices in American Life and Work* (Center for Contemplative Mind in Society, 2004).

13. CMind. (2021). "The Tree of Contemplative Practices [Illustration]." The Center for Contemplative Mind in Society. https://www.contemplativemind.org/practices/tree.

14. Shapiro, Shauna L., Kristen E. Lyons, Richard C. Miller, Britta Butler, Cassandra Vieten, and Philip David Zelazo. "Contemplation in the Classroom: A New Direction for Improving Childhood Education." *Educational Psychol-*

ogy Review 27, no. 1 (2015): 1–30; Mind and Life Education Research Network (MLERN); Richard J. Davidson, John Dunne, Jacquelynne S. Eccles, Adam Engle, Mark Greenberg, Patricia Jennings, et al. "Contemplative Practices and Mental Training: Prospects for American Education." *Child Development Perspectives* 6, no. 2 (2012): 146–53.

15. Duerr, M. *A Powerful Silence*.

16. King-McKenzie, Ethel. "Death and Dying in the Curriculum of Public Schools: Is There a Place?" *Journal of Emerging Knowledge on Emerging Markets* 3, no. 1 (2011): 29.

17. Saint Joseph's University. "Death Education: Preparing Teens for End-of-Life Issues," August 6, 2021. https://www.sju.edu/news/death-education-preparing-teens-end-life-issues.

18. Stover, Kailen. "Teaching Students about Death and Grief." Edutopia. George Lucas Educational Foundation, March 6, 2020. https://www.edutopia.org/article/teaching-students-about-death-and-grief.

19. Talwar, Victoria. "Talking to Children about Death in Educational Settings." In *Children's Understanding of Death: From Biological to Religious Conceptions*, edited by Victoria Talwar, Paul L. Harris, and Michael Schleifer (Cambridge University Press, 2011), 98–115. King-McKenzie, "Death and Dying."

20. Jenkinson, Stephen. *Die Wise: A Manifesto for Sanity and Soul* (North Atlantic Books, 2015).

21. Nunez, Kirsten. "How Eye Gazing May Bring You Closer to Someone Else." Healthline. Healthline Media, October 13, 2020. https://www.healthline.com/health/eye-gazing#eye-contact-psychology.

22. Fullwood, C., and G. Doherty-Sneddon. "Effect of Gazing at the Camera during a Video Link on Recall." *Applied Ergonomics* 37, no. 2 (2006): 167–75. https://doi:10.1016/j.apergo.2005.05.003; Kreysa, H., L. Kessler, and S. R. Schweinberger. "Direct Speaker Gaze Promotes Trust in Truth-Ambiguous Statements." K. Paterson (Ed.). *PLOS ONE* 11, no. 9 (2016): e0162291. https://doi:10.1371/journal.pone.0162291.

23. Myllyneva, Aki, and Jari K. Hietanen. "There Is More to Eye Contact than Meets the Eye." *Cognition* 134 (2015): 100–109; Dumas, Thibaud, Stéphanie Dubal, Yohan Attal, Marie Chupin, Roland Jouvent, Shasha Morel, and Nathalie George. "MEG Evidence for Dynamic Amygdala Modulations by Gaze and Facial Emotions." Edited by Andreas Keil. *PLOS ONE* 8, no. 9 (September 10, 2013): e74145. https://doi.org/10.1371/journal.pone.0074145.

CHAPTER 11

1. Merton, Thomas. *Conjectures of a Guilty Bystander* (Doubleday, 1966).
2. World Health Organization. "International Classification of Diseases, 11th Revision." https://icd.who.int/en (2018); American Psychiatric Association. "Diagnostic and Statistical Manual of Mental Disorders: DSM-5-TR" (2022).

INDEX

Note: Page numbers in *italics* refer to tables and figures. In addition to this printed index, an online index offering flexible filtering and search of every activity and supplement in the book can be accessed at https://tiny.cc/fcindex

About My Name activity, 97
Accept All activity, 155
acceptance, 113, 155. *See also* resilience
achievements, 259–60
acronyms, 124–27, *126*
Acts of Gratitude activity, 200
adverse childhood experiences, 5, 33
Affirmations activity, 201
agreements, 44–47, 62, 90
Altruism activity, 108
Angakkorsuaq, Angaangaq, 258
Angelou, Maya, 33, 131
Animal Groups activity, 106–7
Announcing Well-Being activity, 31

Anonymous Feedback Channels activity, 40–44, *41*
Appreciation Contemplation activity, 199–200
Appreciationships activity, *190*, 190–92, *193*
Aronson, Eliot, 214–15
art activities, 76–77, 171
Ask Three, Then Me activity, 137
assessments: *Plumbing the Well*, 26–31; *Safer Assessment*, 53; standardized, 143–44; *Student Self-Assessment*, 110; for well-being, 3, 31
Atlas of Emotions activity, 197
Aurelius, Marcus, 237

authenticity, 59. *See also* eudaimonia
Auto-Mindfulness activity, 153
awareness of the inner body. *See Interoception* activity
awareness of well-being, 35

Backchannels and Polls activity, 83
Bacon, Francis, 9
barriers to vulnerability, 45
Become activity, 154
Becoming the Pulse activity, 152
belly breaths, 148
belonging, 56. *See also* social well-being
Bergman, Carrie, 239
Best Self activity, 108
Bishop, Orland, 133
Body Literacy activity, 24–25
body scans, 149
Brain Breaks activity, 170
break boxes, 3, 49, 52
Bring Nature In activity, 210–11
bronze achievements, 259
Brown, Brené, 42

Call Me by My True Name activity, 52
Calm Place activity, 152
cards, 263–71
Cards feedback, 50
Caring Adult Connections activity, 64–66
Catching Goodness activity, 66–68, 67
Ceasing practice, *162*
Celebrating Growth and Excellence activity, 108
centerpieces in circles, 60
Cervantes, Miguel de, 127
Character Traits activity, *114*, 137

Chatzky, Jean, 113
check-in prompts, *62–63*
Cherish Other activity, 152
Chinese character for listening, 70, 71
Choice Moments activity, 115–19, 119–22
Choose Acronym activity, 125
Chose Refuge activity, 19–20
circles: *Appreciationships, 190*, 190–92, *193*; capacity of, 59; *Circle Check-Ins,* 57–63, *62–63*; *Circle Energizers,* 229; *Circle Games,* 197–98; *Circle Gazing,* 247; *Circles of Resilience,* 137–38, *138*; *Dancing Circles,* 229; for death dialogues, 244–45; debriefing in, 90; for emotional regulation, 185–86; for eudaimonia, 97; *Fishbowl Circles, 190,* 190–92, *193*; *Restorative Circles,* 136
classroom agreements, 44–47, 62, 90
classroom disruptions, 176
Classroom Ergonomics activity, 229
Clock Watching activity, 154–55
Closing Circle activity, 256–58
Coates, Ta-Nehisi, 87
Cognitive Distortion Scavenger Hunt, 170
cognitive well-being: about, 8, 143–45; immersive states, 164; key messages, 145; self-assessment reflection questions, 29; *Self-Directed Neuroplasticity,* 156–60, *161–62*; *From Semi-Interested to Flow,* 163–68, *166*; supplementaries, 170–73; *Train That Train,* 168–70. *See also Mindfulness Moments Medley*

INDEX

Collaborative Group Skills activity, 83
Coloring Hath Charms activity, 171
Comforting Oneself activity, 201
communication, 84
community, 4, 35, 87, 255. *See also* classroom agreements; social well-being
compassion, 35
conflict resolution, 133–37, *134*
Connect the Dots activity, 171
Contemplative Practices, 238–41, *239*
Content Warnings activity, 52
"CORE" steps, 157–59, *161–62*, 264n17
coronavirus pandemic, 203
Could Be Good, Could Be Bad activity, 127–29
counting breaths, 148
COVID-19, 203
Creativity Is Joy activity, 171
Crossed/Uncrossed activity, 198
Crossing the Streams activity, 154
Csikszentmihalyi, Mihaly, 7, 111, 163, 165
curriculum evolution, 3–4

Dancing Circles, 229
data. *See* Programme for International Student Assessment (PISA)
Dawson, Paul, 64
Death Dialogues, 242–45
debriefing experiences: benefits, 14–15; for cognitive well-being, 155, 159, 168, 169; *Debriefing Anything*, 13–17; for emotional well-being, 188, 192, 195, 196–97; for eudaimonia, 98–99, 102–3, 107; for interoception, 25–26; for physical well-being, 219, 224–25; preparation for, 15; questions for, 14, 15, *16–17*; for resilience, 118, 125, 128, 132, 137; for returning to presence, 20–21; for safety, 43, 47; for social well-being, 61, 67, 73, 74, 77, 79, 81–82; for spiritual well-being, 241, 245, 247, 250; stages, 15–16

Decision Time activity, 171
Deeper Questions activity, 251
Die Wise (Jenkinson), 243
Digital Portfolios activity, 108
Disraeli, Benjamin, 184
domains of well-being, 7–9. *See also* cognitive well-being; emotional well-being; environmental well-being; eudaimonia; social well-being; spiritual well-being
Doorways to Connection activity, 68–70
Doorways to Presence activity, 154
Drawing Breath (or Music) activity, 148
Duerr, Maia, 238, 239

Earth/Eco/Green/Environment activity, 211
Einstein, Albert, 248
Elvish Sleep activity, 229
emojis, 181, 182
Emotional Gift Research activity, 182, 198–99
emotional inquiry process, 182
emotional intelligence (EQ), 177, 178–79
emotional well-being: about, 8, 175–77; *Emotional Journals*, 183; *Emotional Regulation(s)*, 184–86; *Emotional Well-Being Apps*, 199; *Emotion Moments*,

152–53; *E-Motions Scavenger Hunt*, 186–88, *189*; *Feels Wheels*, 180–84, *181*; *Fishbowl Circles*, *190*, 190–92, *193*; *Heartwarming*, 194–95; hedonic treadmill, 177–79; immersive states, 164; key messages, 180; making feelings visible, 36–37; self-assessment reflection questions, 29; *Self-Care/Self-Love Playsheet*, 220–22; supplementaries, 197–201; *Taking Back How Are You?*, 195–97; *Taste of Feeling*, 183

environmental well-being: about, 8; *Earth/Eco/Green/Environment*, 211; key messages, 206; *Nature Immersion*, 208–10; outdoor learning, 203–6, *205*; self-assessment reflection questions, 29; supplementaries, 210–12; *Walk the Talk*, 206–8

EQ (emotional intelligence), 177, 178–79

eudaimonia: about, 8, 85–88, 100; *Animal Groups*, 106–7; emotional well-being and, 179; generativity, 87–88; immersive states, 164; *Inviting Identity*, 93–99; key messages, 88; *MEGA-SMARTER Goal Journeys*, 100–104, *105–6*; *A Question of Purpose*, 88–91, *91–93*; self-assessment reflection questions, 29; supplementaries, 108–10

exercises. *See* physical well-being

Exit Passes activity, 42

Explore, Compare, and Connect activity, 183

eye contact, 245–47

Eyes of Love activity, 151

faint, flop, flag reactions, *121*

F.A.R.M. the Joy, 271

fawn reactions, *121*

feedback, 36, 40–44, *41*, 50, 50–51

Feedback Fades Fear activity, 53

Feeling Cue activity, 152

Feelings Maps activity, 199

Feels Wheels activity, 180–84, *181*

fidget tamers, 49, 60

fight reactions, *120*

Finger Labyrinths activity, 150

Fipps, Lisa, 68

Fishbowl Circles, 106, *190*, 190–92, *193*

Fist to Five feedback, 50

5-4-3-2-1 activity, 155

flexibility, 36

flight reactions, *121*

flow state, 163–68, *166*, 171

Focus Elements activity, 209

followups on feedback, 40, *41*

foraging for food, 209–10

Ford, Ashtyn, 76

Forest Schools programs, 211

Formal Body Meditation activity, 150

Formal Breath Meditation activity, 149

Foshay, Arthur W., 143

Frankl, Viktor, 88

Fredrickson, Barbara, 100

freeze reactions, *120*

Friend to Self activity, 201

From Semi-Interested to Flow activity, 163–68, *166*

furniture in classrooms, 48

Gains and Drains activity, 231–32

gaming comparison, 165

Gandhi, Mahatma, 1

INDEX

Gay, Roxane, 93
gazing activity, 245–47
Geneva wheel, 181
Give a Little Bit activity, 199
"Giving Up" activity, 138
goals. *See* MEGA-SMARTER Goal Journeys
Going Green (Give One, Get One) activity, 211
Going on a Picnic activity, 198
gold achievements, 260
Goleman, Daniel, 47
goodness, 66–68. *See also Seeing and Sharing the Goodness* activity
Go Slow to Go Fast activity, 52–53
governmental innovations, 1
Graham, Linda, 124
gratitude: *Gratitude Lists*, 199; *Gratitude Murals*, 199; *Gratitudinals* activities, 199–200, 269; importance of, 36, 179, 199–200
grit *vs.* resilience, 112
group discussions, 45–46
growth. *See* eudaimonia
Guided Meditation activity, 248–51

habits, 156–57
hand signals for safety, 50, 50–51
Hanson, Rick, 139
Harris, Sydney J., 26
Head, Shoulder, Knees, and Toes . . . and PEN! activity, 233
health care parable, 6–7
heart vocabulary. *See* emotional well-being
Heartwarming activity, 194–95, 268
hedonia. *See* emotional well-being
hedonic treadmill, 177–79

Help Wanted Microlab activity, 129–31, *130*
Hobby Talk activity, 108–9
hope and resilience, 138–39
How Are You? question, 195–97
Human Being or Human Doing? activity, 251
Huppert, Felicia, 55

I am . . . I am not . . . activity, 109
I Like My Neighbor activity, 198
immersive state. *See From Semi-Interested to Flow* activity
Inhabiting Self activity, 25
Inner Body Awareness activity, 150
inner body feelings. *See Interoception* activity
Inner Caring Committee activity, 139
Inside/Outside Circles activity, 83
inspirational postings, 49
integration strategies: about, 9; in cognitive domain, 167, 170; for cognitive well-being, 155, 160; for debriefing, 17; for environmental well-being, 207, 210; for eudaimonia, 91, 99, 103; for interoception, 26; for physical well-being, 217, 225; for refuge, 22; for resilience, 118–19, 125, 128–29, 131, 133; for safety, 43–44, 51; in self-assessment, 29; for social well-being, 74, 82, 83; for spiritual well-being, 241, 245; for well-being, 183–84, 192, 258
intellectual health. *See* cognitive well-being
Intense Presence activity, 151
Interacting 1:1 activity, 83

Interbeing through Gazing activity, 245–47
Interoception activity: as awareness of inner body, 18; card for, 266; emotional well-being and, 179, 182; for feedback, 50; *Inquiring Within*, 22–26
Inviting Identity activity, 93–99
"I" Statements activity, 135
"Is there more?" option, 73, 74

Jenkinson, Stephen, 243
Jennings, Herbert, 111
Jigsaw Accountabilities Group activity, 214–18
journals, 183
joy farming, 158–59, *161*
joyfulness, 36
Joy Jar activity, 200
Junto wheel, 180
Just Do It activity, 153
Just Feel awareness, 149
Just Hear activity, 151–52
Just See activity, 151

Kaling, Mindy, 223
Kendi, Ibram, 34
Kessler, Rachael, 235
Keyes, Corey L. M., 7
keywords, 261–62
Kierkegaard, Søren, 13
Kihaya proverb, 4
kind awareness, 201
kindness to oneself, 194–95
King-McKenzie, Ethel, 242
kintohpatatin, 70
Kiyosaki, Robert, 185
Kornfield, Jack, 78
Krishnamurti, Jiddu, 208

labeling activities: for cognitive well-being, 154, *161–62*; for emotional well-being, 183, 200; *Unlabeling*, 110
Ladder of Student Participation, 109
last words, 256–57
Learning Circles, 171–72
learning united with well-being, 255–58
Le Guin, Ursula K., 85–88
Lennon, John, 237
Lifeline Graphs, 131–33
lifeplay activities: about, 10; for checking into self, 20; for cognitive well-being, 155, 159, 167–68, 170; for debriefing, 17; for emotional well-being, 184, 186, 188, 195, 197; for environmental well-being, 210; for eudaimonia, 91, 99, 102; for interoception, 26; for physical well-being, 217, 219; for resilience, 118, 125, 131, 136; for social well-being, 68, 73–74; for spiritual well-being, 241, 245, 247, 251
Life Support activity, 53
lighting suggestions, 49
listening skills: *Just Hear*, 151–52; *Listen to Silence*, 152; *Mindful Listening*, 70–74, *71*, 147
Love Letters to Self activity, 109, 268
Lovell, Jim, 80
Love Song to Self, 200, 268
Love Text to Self, 201, 268
Loving Containers activity, 47–49

Macy, Joanna, 203
magical teaching/learning moments (MTLMs), 14, 16, 197

INDEX

maintenance of agreements, 46–47
Making the Invisible Visible activity, 36–37, *50*, 50–51
Mandela, Nelson, 66
Mapping Me activity, 109
massage activities, 231
McLaren, Karla, 115, 175, 187
meaning. *See* eudaimonia
Media Ain't Social activity, 83
meditation, guided, 248–51
MEGA-SMARTER *Goal Journeys*, 100–104, *105–6*
MEGA well-being, 86–87
Mendel, Gregor, 100
Mental Health and Mindfulness Apps, 172
mental health of children, 5–7. *See also* cognitive well-being; emotional well-being
Merton, Thomas, 66, 253
Metatawabin, Edmund, 70
microlabs. *See Help Wanted Microlab* activity
mindfulness: *Auto-Mindfulness* activity, 153; emotional well-being and, 179; *Mindful Dialogue*, 84, 271; *Mindful Eating*, 230; *Mindful Listening*, 70–74, *71*, 147, 267; *Mindful Moments* card, 265; *Mindful Sip/Bite* activity, 150; *Mindful Talking*, 153; *Nature Immersion*, 209; *Walking Mindfulness* activity, 153–54. *See also* Mindfulness Moments Medley
Mindfulness Moments Medley: about, 145–47; benefits, 139, 146–47; *Breath Moments*, 148–49; *Emotion Moments*, 152–53; *Feel Moments*, 149–50; *Hear Moments*, 151–52; *Mixed Moments*, 152–53. *See Moments*, 151
Mingle Bingo, 74–75, 76
minorities, 33–35
modeling practice, 21
More Than One Story activity, 109
MTLMs (magical teaching/learning moments), 14, 16, 197
Mystery Box activity, 150

Name It to Tame It activity, 200
Name Your Move activity, 233
natural world, 204–6. *See also* environmental well-being
Nature Immersion activity, 208–10
Near, Far, and All activity, 151
N.E.A.T. activities, 230–31, 270
negativity, 5–7, 159–60, *161–62*
neuroplasticity, 179
Nisbet, Elizabeth, 204
non-governmental organizations' innovations, 1
non-sequential sharing, 61, 90, 97
non-verbal feedback, *50*, 50–51
Norman-Murch, Trudi, 56
Notice for the First Time activity, 151

1, 2, 3, 4 activity, 232–33
One Deep Breath a Day practice, 148
oneness with others, 253
1:1 Check-in activity, 43
Online Surveys, 43
Opening Hope activity, 138–39
Outdoor Classrooms project, 211
outdoor learning, 203–6, *205*. *See also* environmental well-being
Outside the Box activity, 212
Over and Under activity, 233

Palmer, Parker, 218
Partner Drawing activity, 76–77
Partner Lifelines card, 265
peacefulness, 36. *See also* spirituality of RWA
Peace Paths activity, 136
personal agency, 21
Phone Feels activity, 152–53
physical well-being: about, 8, 213–14; key messages, 214; *Physical Well-Being Apps*, 231; *Puzzling Out Wellness with Jigsaw Accountabilities Group*, 214–18; self-assessment reflection questions, 30; *Self-Care/Self-Love Playsheets*, 218–19, 220–22; *Sleep Hygiene Lab*, 223–25, 226–28; supplementaries, 229–33
Pillar Quizzes activity, 231
PISA (Programme for International Student Assessment), 2, 144
Plantastic activity, 172
Plumbing the Well activity, 26–31, 29–30
Plutchik, Robert, 180, *181*
Portrait of Identities activity, 98
positive psychology, 5–7
pre-brief activities, 14
Pretending to Be Funny activity, 200
Programme for International Student Assessment (PISA), 2, 144
prompts: for circles, 60–62, *62–63*, 256–58; for eudaimonia activities, 97, 99; for mindful listening, 19, 70–74. *See also* debriefing experiences
pronunciation of student names, 52
proverbs, 129
public broadcasting of wellness tips, 31

Puzzling Out Wellness activity, 214–18

questions: for circles, 60–62, *62–63*, 258; for debriefing experiences, 14, 15, *16–17*; of living, 12; *Question of Purpose*, 88–91, *91–93*, 269; *Repairing (Almost) Anything*, 133–37, *134*; for self-assessment, 29–30; for thumballs, 82; *True or Not?*, 161

racial bias, 34–35, 214–15
Ray, Amit, 206, 237
Receiving Vibes activity, 153
referrals, 22, 38–39
Refuge activity, 17–22, 24, 147
relationships. *See* social well-being
religion, 236. *See also* spiritual well-being
Remen, Rachel Naomi, 12
Repairing (Almost) Anything activity, 133–37, *134*
Reshaping, Reframing, Redirecting practice, *162*
resilience: about, 8; *Choice Moments*, 115–19, *119–22*; *Circles of Resilience*, 137–38, *138*; *Could Be Good, Could Be Bad*, 127–29; *Help Wanted Microlab*, 129–31, *130*; key messages, 115; *Lifeline Graphs*, 131–33; *Repairing (Almost) Anything*, 133–37, *134*; safety in, 118–19, 125, 128, 131, 133, 137; self-assessment questions, 30; supplementaries, 137–41; *Traits of Resilience*, 113–15, *114*, 130, 140; as universal, 111–13; *Using Life to Free Yourself*, 123–27, *126*

INDEX

Resilientences, 139. *See also Watched Words* activity
response-ability: about, 116–17; *Choice Moments*, 115–19, *119–22*; continuum of, *122*; emotional well-being and, 179; *Using Life to Free Yourself*, 123–27, *126*
responsiveness, 36
restoration: questions for, 15; *Restorative Circles*, 136; *Restorative Talks*, 135. *See also* debriefing experiences; *Repairing (Almost) Anything* activity
Returning activity, 19
Revealing the Target activity, 53
Rewilding activity, 212
Rock, Paper, Scissors Grand Tournament, 233
Ruiz, Don Miguel, 22
Rumi, 256
Ruskin, John, 186
Ryff, Carol D., 7

Safer Assessment activity, 53
safety: about, 8, 33–35; *Anonymous Feedback Channels*, 40–44, *41*; *Classroom Agreements*, 44–47; debriefing strategies, 16–17; in final circles, 257; interoception, 23–24; key messages, 39; *Loving Containers*, 47–49; *Making the Invisible Visible*, 36–37, 50, 50–51; qualities of safer human beings, 35–39; refuge activities and, 21–22; for resilience, 118–19, 125, 128, 131, 133, 137; in self-assessment, 28–29, *30*; sharing information with school administration, 44; supplementaries, 52–53; trust and, 47
safety issues in activities: for cognitive well-being, 147, 160, 168, 169–70; for emotional well-being, 183, 188, 192, 197; for environmental well-being, 208, 209–10; for eudaimonia, 90–91, 99, 101, 107; for physical well-being, 217–18, 225; for social well-being, 61–62, 65, 67, 69, 74, 77, 79, 82; for spiritual well-being, 241, 243–44, 251
Safety Nets activity, 53
Sahib, Bhai, 123
Salzberg, Sharon, 194
Santorelli, Saki, 240
Sápa, Heháka, 190
scavenger hunts, 186–88, *189*
school administration, 38–39, 44, 255–56
schoolwide extensions: about, 9; as closings, 258; for cognitive well-being, 155; for emotional well-being, 192; for environmental well-being, 208; for eudaimonia, 103; for physical well-being, 217, 225; for refuge, 22; for resilience, 137; for safety, 44; for social well-being, 66, 68, 69–70
Schwartz, Jeffrey M., 156
Seeing and Sharing the Goodness activity, 78–79, 88
See the Sky activity, 151
segregation in schools, 214–15
SEL (social-emotional learning), 57, 176–77
self-assessments: involving students in, 3, 31; *Plumbing the Well*

activity, 26–31, 29–30; *Student Self-Assessment*, 110
Self-Care/Love Acronyms activity, 232, 266
Self-Care/Self-Love Playsheets, 218–19, 220–22
Self-Compassion Practices, 21, 200–201
Self-Directed Neuroplasticity activity, 156–60, *161–62*, 264n17
Self-Love Acronym card, 266
Self Massage activity, 231
self-regulation, 21
Self-Talk Team Turnaround activity, 139–40
Seligman, Martin, 7, 177
semi-anonymous feedback, 50, *50–51*
Senegalese proverb, 129
sensory experiences, 22–23, 209. *See also Interoception* activity
sequential rounds in circles, 61
seven-eleven breathing, 148
shareable cards, 10, 11, 255
shining inner circles, 46
Siegel, Dan, 200
silver achievements, 259–60
single-celled organisms, 111
Skin Breathing activity, 153
Sleep Hygiene Lab, 223–25, *226–28*, 270
SMARTER Eco-Action, 210
Snowballs activity, 42–43
Sobel, David, 204
social-emotional learning (SEL), 57, 176–77
social media challenges, 83
Social Progress Index, 1
social regulation, 185
social well-being: about, 8, 55–57, 255; *Caring Adult Connections*, 64–66; *Catching Goodness*, 66–68, *67*; *Circle Check-Ins*, 57–63, *62–63*; *Doorways to Connection*, 68–70; key messages, 57; *Mindful Listening*, 70–74, *71*; *Mingle Bingo*, 74–75, *76*; *Partner Drawing*, 76–77; *Seeing and Sharing the Goodness*, 78–79; self-assessment questions, 30; *Self-Care/Self-Love Playsheet*, 220–22; supplementaries, 83–84; *Thumball Sharing*, 80–82, *82*
Sole Focus activity, 150
Soothing Touch activity, 150
Speakeasy Jigsaws, 84
spiritual well-being: about, 8, 235–38; *Contemplative Practices*, 238–41, *239*; *Death Dialogues*, 242–45; *Interbeing through Gazing*, 245–47; key messages, 238; self-assessment reflection questions, 30; *Self-Care/Self-Love Playsheet*, 220–22; supplementaries, 251; *Unselfing*, 248–51
Square Breathing activity, 149
Squeeze and Release activity, 150
Story of My Life activity, 97
stressful events. *See Choice Moments* activity
Stress Signals activity, 140
Stretches and Exercises, 231
Student Choice and Voice activity, 109–10
student feedback, 36, 40–44, *41*
Student Self-Assessment, 110
student-staff relationships, 64–66
success, 254
Sustainable Development Goals, 1

INDEX

Take a Stand activity, 232
Take Five Movement Breaks activity, 232–33
Taking Back How Are You? activity, 195–97
Taking Refuge activity, 17–22, 24, 147, 264
Talk about Anything card, 264
talking pieces, 60, 61, 62, 90, 108
Tanzanian proverb, 4
Taste of Feeling activity, 183
T-Chart activity, 128
technology, 175
Thank Not Bank activity, 200
"*That's Me!*" activity, 110
Thích Nhất Hạnh, 145, 245, 246
Thoreau, Henry David, 5
Thought Journaling, 172
Three Filters activity, 84, *162*
Three Refuges activity, 19
Three Reminders activity, 20
Three What's activity, 140–41
Thumball Sharing activity, 80–82, *82*
Thumbs feedback, 50
Tone Down activity, 152
Toss Across activity, 229
Touchstone activity, 150
Tracing Fingers activity, 149
Train That Train activity, 168–70
Traits of Resilience activity, 113–15, *114*, 130, 140
transcendence. See spiritual well-being
Tree of Contemplative Practices, 239, *239*, 240–41
True or Not? questions, *161*
trust, levels of, 37–38, 42
2SLGBTQ+ teens, 33–34

union. See spiritual well-being
United Nations, 1

Unlabeling activity, 110
Unselfing activity, 248–51
Unstuck Posters activity, 141
upstream parable, 6–7
Useful or Not? labeling, *161*
Using Life to Free Yourself activity, 123–27, *126*, 159

Value Lines activity, 172
VIA Character Institute, 31
Virtues Vocab activity, 31
visibility. See *Making the Invisible Visible* activity
Visible Random Groups activity, 84
vulnerability, 36, 42

Wakinyan, Chief (Dave Yakima), 57
Walk and Roll activity, 212
Walking Mindfulness activity, 153–54
Walk the Talk activity, 206–8, 267
wall space, 48–49
Watched Words activity, 173
Welcome Graffiti activity, 53
well-being: about, 9–10, 254–55; classroom approaches to, 10–11, 255–56; *Closing Circle*, 256–58; *Debriefing Anything*, 13–17; *Plumbing the Well*, 26–31, *29–30*; supplementaries, 31; *Taking Refuge*, 17–22, 24, 147
Wellness Wednesdays, 3
Well Seated activity, 31
We Wall activity, 96–97
wholeness, 253
whole-village approach, 4
Williams, Terry Tempest, 18
Wise and Loving Mind practice, *162*
Wishing Well activity, 84

Words of Feeling activity, 201
World Happiness Report, 1
World Health Organization, 213

X-Ray Ears activity, 152

Yakima, Dave (Chief Wakinyan), 57
Yin Yang activity, 128

Zen parable, 242
Zola, Irving, 6

ABOUT THE AUTHOR

Jeff Catania was a computer engineer briefly, then a teacher longingly. Having two left brains, for decades he led K–12 district programs in eLearning, information technology and mathematics. On discovering his right brain, heart, and soul, he launched mindfulness, restorative practices, and well-being initiatives, facilitating professional development across North America.

Jeff is a contributing author to *Rebooting Assessment* (with Damian Cooper, IBPA Ben Franklin Gold Medal winner for best book in education), *Talk about Assessment* (with Damian Cooper), and *The Joy of X: Mathematics Teaching in Grades 7–12* (with Shirley Dalrymple and George Gadanidis). He now enjoys farm life with his mate Barb, facilitates support groups for betrayed partners, and leads learning experiences to deepen peace, joy, and love.

Visit Jeff at https://alove.ca.

www.ingramcontent.com/pod-product-compliance
Lightning Source LLC
Chambersburg PA
CBHW022009300426
44117CB00005B/104